Living with
HALF A HEART

A Mother's Guide to Navigating Fontan Surgery

LIBBY ANDREW

First published by Ultimate World Publishing 2019
Copyright © 2019 Libby Andrew

ISBN

Paperback - 978-1-925884-91-3
Ebook - 978-1-925884-92-0

Libby Andrew has asserted her right under the Copyright, Designs and Patents Act 1988 to be identified as the author of this work. The information in this book is based on the author's experiences and opinions. The publisher specifically disclaims responsibility for any adverse consequences, which may result from use of the information contained herein. Permission to use information has been sought by the author. Any breaches will be rectified in further editions of the book.

All rights reserved. No part of this publication may be reproduced, stored in or introduced into a retrieval system, or transmitted in any form, or by any means (electronic, mechanical, photocopying, recording or otherwise) without the prior written permission of the author. Any person who does any unauthorised act in relation to this publication may be liable to criminal prosecution and civil claims for damages. Enquiries should be made through the publisher.

Cover design: Ultimate World Publishing
Layout and typesetting: Ultimate World Publishing
Editor: James Salmon

Ultimate World Publishing
Diamond Creek,
Victoria Australia 3089
www.writeabook.com.au

TESTIMONIALS

A great read for parents at any stage in the pathway to Fontan. Libby's writing style is direct and informative. Her comments on the necessary partnership between medical carers and families is a great takeaway.

David S. Winlaw
Vivienne and Ross Hobson
Professor in Paediatric Cardiac Disease
The University of Sydney
Faculty of Medicine and Health, The Children's Hospital at Westmead, Heart Centre for Children

A great resource to help support caregivers of kids with complex congenital heart disease navigate through the storm. We called our Fontan Dance "Thomas Turbulence" because it sure was a bumpy ride.

Kelly Ryan, mum to Thomas. Fontan completion performed by Dr Orr at Westmead Children's Hospital, January 2018.

Thank you for sharing your experiences, an open and honest account of your family's journey through the early years of CHD and Fontan surgery. Your story is a valuable, practical resource for other families who are new to the CHD world.

Anne Maree Maher, Midwife

I first met Libby at a catch up for families who have children with heart conditions. I was 25 weeks pregnant with a child with a severe heart defect and the world felt uncertain and cloudy. Libby introduced me to her son Daniel and together they gave me so much hope for my little boy's future. I'm so grateful that Libby is extending her ability to provide hope and information like she did to our family to other families by sharing her journey and this book. A must read for all families of children with severe heart defects.

Mel Clode, Charlie's mum

Touchingly honest and forthright, I thank Libby for giving us a window into her (and Daniel's) journey, and casting light for others on a similar journey. She writes with a reassuring calm that is sure to help parents navigating CHD.

Dr Catherine McDonald, Osteopath.

An invaluable guide for someone seeking more information about the unexpected and unpredictable journey of having a baby with CHD.

Rowena Blewitt, mum to Harper.

CONTENTS

Testimonials iii
Dedication.. vii
Trigger Warning ix
Introduction xi
Chapter 1: The diagnosis 1
Chapter 2: 20 weeks to go 11
Chapter 3: The F words.. 21
Chapter 4: The variety of hospital stays and visits......... 29
Chapter 5: Hospital provisions..................................... 43
Chapter 6: Pulmonary Artery Banding or shunt........... 49
Chapter 7: Bidirectional Glenn Shunt 65
Chapter 8: Preparation for Fontan and Fontan Surgery 75
Chapter 9: Recovering from Fontan Surgery 81
Chapter 10: Wrapping up and getting ready 89
Conclusion: A lifelong commitment to your baby
    and their CHD 95
Retreat Pages.. 101
Glossary... 109
About the Author... 111
Acknowledgements.. 113
"Half a Heart" Facebook Group 115

DEDICATION

To the parents, the families and all children suffering a broken heart; I hope this helps.

Disclaimer

The information contained within this book is for general information only and has been written from a mother's perspective. The purpose is to provide information and support to families. This information is not intended as a substitute for professional medical advice. Please always seek the advice of your baby's cardiologist or any other medical professional on your team.

TRIGGER WARNING

Some of the topics within the pages of this book are confronting. Congenital Heart Disease (CHD) and the suffering caused to your baby can also be confronting.

This suffering has the potential to affect your entire family in various ways.

Diagnosis of a CHD can be a very emotional time, particularly for pregnant mothers.

Some of the content within these pages may trigger a negative response in a reader (e.g panic attack).

Please be alert to your responses and take a break from reading, put the book away or skip a chapter if this happens to you. Go gently.

INTRODUCTION

If you are a mum carrying a precious unborn baby with an imperfect heart, I am here to offer you hope. In July 2013, at 20 week's gestation, my unborn son Daniel was diagnosed with a complex heart defect. Since then, I've kept my notes and Daniel's records in the hopes of compiling a practical handbook to help guide the mums who will follow in search of information about congenital heart disease (CHD) and Fontan Surgery. This is the book that I was unable to find while preparing myself for the birth of a child with a CHD.

In Australia in 2019, eight babies are born every day with some form of a heart defect, four babies die of a CHD or heart defect every week, and CHD is the leading cause of death in infants under the age of one. If I can assist in raising the awareness of these facts and in fundraising dollars for future research, I will have achieved another two goals.

Most people are not aware of these facts until, like me and now you, they are confronted with the decision of whether or not to terminate their unborn child diagnosed with a CHD. Only you can decide if termination is the right option for you. This is a terrifying experience and it's not easy, but for Daniel and possibly your child, there may be many wonderful years following their rugged entry into life.

Congenital Heart Disease (CHD) refers to heart problems in unborn babies, as opposed to Coronary Heart Disease which mainly affects adults. The CHD that your baby now carries may go hand-in-hand with the Fontan Surgery. Your doctor may have diagnosed your baby with one or more heart conditions. Daniel was eventually diagnosed with a Tricuspid Atresia, among other complications including Dextrocardia, Congenitally Corrected Transposition of the Great Vessels, an Atrial Septal Defect (ASD) and an Ventricular Septal Defect (VSD). His treatment included three delicate stages of Fontan surgery, which will be described in the later chapters of this book.

Fontan Surgery is a palliative treatment for a range of complex heart diseases in babies and is often the only option for children born at the upper end of the defect spectrum. This means that the Fontan is not a cure. It can be very difficult to accept that your baby's heart condition may not be able to be fixed. What I can tell you from my own experience is that this does not mean that your baby cannot enjoy the life that you are about to provide. At the time of Daniel's second ultrasound at 20 weeks gestation, I was advised to terminate the pregnancy because my baby would most likely not survive. The doctor told me that "this baby would not fit into any person's lifestyle". As this book goes to print, Daniel is a rambunctious, happy six-year-old boy enjoying life to the maximum.

A little piece of advice that was shared with me upon entry into this amazing and excruciating congenital heart world – it's often a case of taking two steps backwards before you can take one step forward. I will refer to this advice from this point on as the "Fontan Dance". One guarantee in this new adventure is that you will experience setbacks. These can hit like a sledgehammer and take you to a place of unknown stress and hardship. However, at the equally amazing opposite end of that spectrum there is gratitude, appreciation and life's beauty that you, like me, may get to experience.

You are about to enter a whole new world where you will meet some amazing professionals who can provide you with the advice necessary

INTRODUCTION

for you to make the best decisions for your baby. Here are a few quick pointers to help you start your journey:

- You will have lots of questions. Grab yourself a pad and pen and start writing them down now so you won't need to remember them on appointment day. Don't hold back and don't be too afraid to ask the questions that frighten or confront you. Doctors are pretty good at drawing diagrams too, so don't be shy to ask for these and a future long-term plan. Remember that plans can and do change upon the birth of your baby.

- If you don't feel like you have made a good connection with your midwife, doctor, surgeon or paediatric cardiologist, remember that you can seek another referral to find the right fit for you. The same goes with the hospital, find the best fit even if that means extra travel. It is important that you feel comfortable and have faith in the people on your team and the services they provide. My advice is to place your trust in their abilities and take their advice, these professionals come with a wealth of experience and knowledge and obviously love what they do.

- Consider obtaining a voice recording application on your mobile phone or other electronic device. Ask the doctor or specialist prior to your meeting if it's okay to record the discussion so you can review it later, research any new terms, share the content or transcript with your family, and to keep as a record. Lots of new words and terminology are coming your way.

- Listen to the advice of your doctors, midwife, specialists and family, but most of all, listen to your own heart and always go with your gut instinct. There will be options, even if some suggest there aren't, and don't let anyone pressure you into doing anything that doesn't feel right. It's okay to say no and okay to ask for some more time to think things over.

- If you start to feel overwhelmed, at any time, be mindful of how you are feeling. Try not to panic and implement the strategies that work best for you to remain calm. Some days will be harder than others. Fontan Surgery is a lifelong commitment even after the first three stages are completed. Ongoing and annual checks will be required at the very minimum.

- There is a wonderful heart community in this country and worldwide. New friends and families await you. The Australian and New Zealand Fontan Registry (ANZFR) is leading the way in the registration and collection of data on Fontan patients in our country. Joining this magnificent team can be equally as beautiful as it is heart-crushing. The ANZFR is pioneering a pathway forward for all children in this country with single ventricle circulation, and their families and teams too.

- Technology and research is improving every year. Babies and children suffering from a range of CHD's are living longer than ever before.

Please read this handbook at a pace that you can handle. Remember to be gentle with yourself as you are now a precious "Heart Mum" and more than likely, soon to be arriving towards the end of your second trimester. If at any point within this book you feel overwhelmed by the content, please take a break from reading. Consider going for a walk, get some fresh air and gentle exercise, make a cup of tea, say a prayer, call a friend, take a bath or skip a chapter if it's all too much for you right now. Put the book away and come back to it when you need to.

I have broken the book into logical and chronological steps towards achieving Fontan circulation. Be mindful of where you are at right at this moment and just breathe. Towards the back of this book I have included a "retreat page", so when all else fails go to page 99 for a short prayer, a poem or an inspirational message. I hope this helps.

INTRODUCTION

Also located at the back end of this handbook is a glossary written in "Libby's words" to try to help you become familiar with some of the terms that might be new to you and their meanings. I hope the glossary can make understanding and referencing a little easier than it was in my experience.

1.

THE DIAGNOSIS

Ultrasounds provide amazing information and imagery. The technology is progressing rapidly with 3D ultrasounds now able to detect more and more birth defects prior to birth. However, just remember that this technology is not foolproof and sometimes the information gathered can be incorrect. In these cases, people may receive a false-negative result that failed to detect an existing defect or a false-positive result that detected a defect that wasn't really there.

Ultrasounds, at the time of going to print, are still conducted by imperfect human beings, real people who will add to the experience of this day. When you front up for the 20-week ultrasound you will find a highly trained health professional, either a sonographer or radiographer depending on their training and qualifications. The purpose of this ultrasound is to examine fetal development.

When you booked in for the 20-week ultrasound, you would have been given instructions. These should have included a specified quantity of water required to be consumed prior to your arrival and testing. You should refrain from emptying your bladder until the scanning is complete.

During the scanning, the sonographer holds a small device called an ultrasound probe in one hand. Their other hand is used to operate the computer and electronic equipment that takes images and measurements of your baby. Gel will be applied to the probe to make it easy to glide this instrument across your baby bump. The gel can get messy and is sticky, and sometimes it can get onto your clothing. It might also feel cold on your skin. During the scanning you should be able to see the images of your baby on a nearby monitor.

Some operators will talk to you while others prefer silence to concentrate.

Around the time of your 20-week scan, your baby's heart is about the size of your thumb nail. The majority of parents arrive excitedly on this day hoping to identify the sex of their baby, but sometimes, additional and unwelcome information becomes apparent too. This day can be a "life changer". If a serious problem was detected in your unborn baby and I am guessing that this may be the case if you are holding this book, your news on this day was shocking and unexpected.

During the scan, the sonographer conducts a number of tests on the baby. He or she is checking the development of the brain, heart, limbs, kidneys, face, bones, blood vessels, umbilical cord etc. The scan usually takes less than an hour, depending on how accommodating your baby decides to be at the time, and whether or not the sonographer is aware of your baby's condition.

If the sonographer detects any problem, it's unlikely they will discuss it with you during the scanning as this information needs to be reviewed by the appropriate professionals before disclosure. Once the scanning is complete, the sonographer wipes the gel off your belly (or you can do so yourself) and you'll finally be allowed to empty your bladder. The sonographer then collates and saves the images, and these findings are discussed with a doctor prior to the report being written. This report

THE DIAGNOSIS

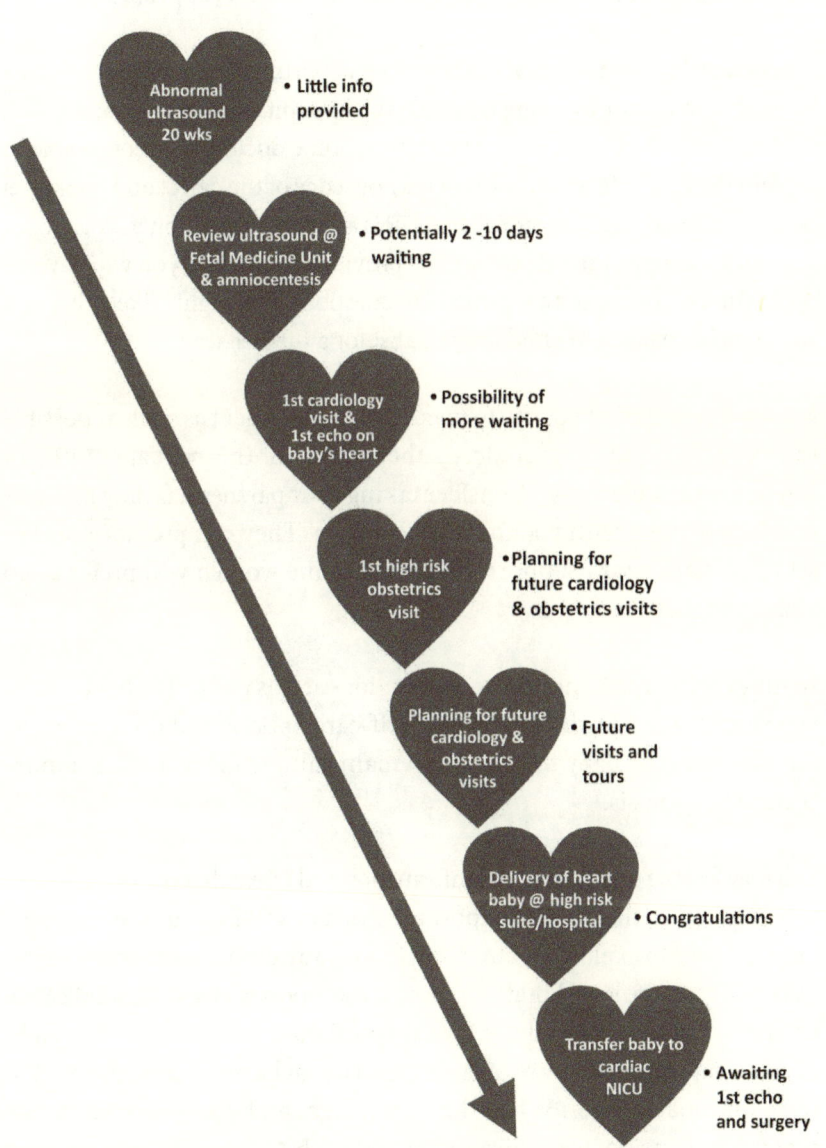

An anticipated journey from 1st ultrasound to 1st surgery

is forwarded to your own doctor and it is normal for you to leave this appointment with very little information about the results of this scan. Talk to the operator and ask any questions when it is appropriate.

If a problem has been detected, at the earliest opportunity, you will be contacted by your own doctor to arrange a follow-up appointment. Some doctors will try to explain the report and the contents. Some doctors will not be able to explain the issues depending on their knowledge of the defect and their level of experience in CHD. Remember, a GP is a general practitioner, not a heart specialist. A copy of the report will be provided to you and you will have an opportunity to discuss any immediate questions. It is highly likely that you will then be referred to another specialist for a further scan.

My suggestion is that you try to make this appointment as soon as possible to relieve the build-up of anxiety – the waiting for this next appointment can be tough. Take it easy. Consider taking your partner, a family member or a friend along with you for this next scan. They can provide another set of ears and extra support. Of course, some women will prefer to go alone and that's okay too.

In my experience, it's normal to feel anxious at this point. Try not to allow your anxiety to snowball. Use your self-care options and do what's best for you and your baby to help you remain calm while you await a more accurate diagnosis.

You may feel the urge to seek out information and research some of the terms/words raised in the original report provided to you by your GP. You may have the urge to explore Doctor Google, visit various internet and hospital websites, go to the local library, or discuss the report with a friend, colleague or family member. My advice is that you should do whatever feels right for you, but please be aware of and careful about harmful misinformation from informal sources. When the time is right and you have an accurate diagnosis, your doctor will provide you with the specific information required. Too much information too soon can be overwhelming. Being drip-fed this information is sometimes a better option.

THE DIAGNOSIS

Fontan Surgery is a three-staged process. Some parents will prefer to read up on one stage at a time to try to get their heads around the amazing and mind-boggling method in which the heart can be "re-plumbed". Other mums' may prefer to read about the entire three-stages at once. Talk to your doctor and ask for their advice. A mountain of material regarding Fontan Surgery exists. Remember that this information can be totally irrelevant and frightening if you haven't yet received a clear diagnosis about your baby's condition.

If you have a partner and they have the urge to conduct research into Fontan Surgery and you don't, make sure you discuss this difference prior to engaging in any discussion and sharing of any information between you. Remember, each person involved will be having their own unique experience, and each person's experience is valid, even that of expecting grandparents. Good communication is key to surviving the journey ahead.

Aside from your pregnancy, many other practical things may need attention in preparation for the next scan. If you find yourself having to travel interstate or a long distance for this next scan, consider checking your vehicle and arranging transport. Ensure you have clear instructions from the referring clinic in order to arrive at the specified location on time. Remember to ask where to park and about facilities at the hospital like meals, sibling care, etc. Don't forget about the multitude of other requirements in preparation for this day (e.g. the needs of older siblings, their transport to and from school, meals, sporting commitments, food for yourself upon arriving home after a long and stressful day, pets, security, etc.). Every pregnancy will be different and some mums will have more challenging needs and responsibilities compared to others. Good planning and being organised will help to relieve any extra stress for this day.

If you are travelling to this next ultrasound, you could use the time in the car to review the list of questions you've made thus far. Pack your favourite music, listen to a podcast or speaker that you enjoy, and provide whatever distraction you need to best prepare yourself. Remember to keep hydrated too and try to get into the practice of carrying drinking water with you wherever you go.

Arriving for this next scan will be similar to the previous one. Drink the required quantity of water specified, take health care cards, identification, previous doctors reports and anything else you feel might be relevant. Don't forget your notepad, support person and recording device. In addition to your partner, you may wish to take your mum, sister or friend.

This scan will be similar to the others however the room may be larger with additional equipment. The examination starts when the lights are dim. The cardiologist or operator may ask for complete silence while they concentrate. This silence can be tough to get through so remember your calming techniques and meditations. Immediately after the scanning, the doctor will discuss their findings with you. Remember to ask permission to audio record this conversation if this is your preference.

At this time, you may also be offered an amniocentesis. This is a separate test which can identify genetic diseases and chromosomal abnormalities. It would usually be conducted at the same time as your scan (or even offered at the previous one). The results of this test can take up to a week depending on where you live and access to required laboratories. During this test, approximately two tablespoons of amniotic fluid is carefully extracted from the amniotic sac within the uterus, and the fetal cells are removed from the fluid to be tested. This test, like most others, comes with risks and may or may not identify further complications. Ask the doctor why he would like you to have the test. Don't rush into your decision, weigh up the pros and cons and go with your gut instinct. There are risks – there always are.

The doctor at this point will give you the best advice available in his or her experience. He or she may also suggest a further scan by another operator/cardiologist. The suggestion of terminating the pregnancy may also be raised at this point. Breathe, trust your gut and take your time. Remember, you are in good hands.

If the doctor has suggested that your baby will require Fontan Surgery, you may have received a diagnosis including one, two, three, or even more

THE DIAGNOSIS

defects (this is normal for Fontan babes). The common diagnoses that qualify for the Fontan include (but are not limited to):

- Tricuspid Atresia
- Pulmonary Atresia with underdeveloped right ventricle (some sub-types)
- Double Inlet Left Ventricle
- Double Outlet Right Ventricle (some sub-types)
- Hypoplastic Left Heart Syndrome (HLHS) and Hypoplastic Right Heart Syndrome (HRHS)
- A range of other heart defects that cannot be fixed by other means to achieve a two-ventricle circulation.

At this point you are probably feeling scared, worried, even physically sick. Some parents choose to seek another opinion from another trained cardiologist. At some point after receiving this information you will make your own decision about whether to proceed with this pregnancy or not.

Some questions that you might consider at this time:

- In the short term, what does this condition mean?
- What surgery will be required?
- How many of these types of surgery do you conduct each year?
- What is your experience with this condition?
- Can you provide me with written information about this condition?
- Is there a fact sheet provided by the hospital?
- Where would I best find information about this condition?
- Is my baby going to be okay?
- What is the life expectancy for my baby?
- What should I expect might happen?
- What are the most likely complications?
- What is the time frame for surgery?
- When will the first surgery most likely be?

- How long might we be in hospital for each surgery?
- Will my baby enjoy a normal life? Or will this condition be limiting? If so, in what anticipated ways?
- What other problems can arise with this condition?
- What are the risks of surgery?
- Can I return to work following birth? If so, when would I need more time off? What would you expect at this stage?
- Will I be able to breastfeed my baby?
- Will my baby require any special diets?
- Are there any costs?
- What is your advice to me?
- Can you suggest any other options that I might consider?
- What is the first thing you might suggest I do now?
- What support is available for me and my family?
- In the long term, what does this condition mean for my baby and my family?
- What are the expected long-term results?
- Will there be lifelong problems that I need to consider for my baby?

Remember, the specialists are human too. They will give you the best advice in their experience. Some people have strong opinions and will not hold back in sharing these with you. My advice is to take your time and look after yourself and your baby.

Here are some other things to consider at the time of receiving the diagnosis:

If you are a working mum or are planning to return to the workforce post-delivery, you may need to make an appointment with your Human Resources team to discuss leave policies, wages and your full range of entitlements. Formulate a return to work plan if you are heading down this road so that you are aware of any time limits that may apply. Some families will unexpectedly spend long periods in hospital, others will be discharged shortly after birth, and some will need to go back and forth. No two journeys are the same, just remember the Fontan Dance (two steps backwards before gaining any forward momentum at times)!

THE DIAGNOSIS

If you have the energy, try to make some precious extra time to spend with your partner. It is important for you both to stay well connected along this journey and communicate. It is important for you to relax too.

If you are inclined, you may also like to seek out support from pregnant womens' groups. Some hospitals may even have mentors in place to assist you with your needs. HeartKids Australia is an amazing association providing support, advice and much more to families of kids with CHD. The hospital social workers and nurses will guide you to their offices within the hospital and provide contact details. Alternatively, google HeartKids Australia and search for other support groups to obtain more information. You will be amazed at just how much support is available to you if you seek it. You can also visit my website www.halfaheart.com.au where you will find useful information, links and suggested resources. You're welcome to email me with any queries and I will do my best to help.

There are also a multitude of Facebook groups for various heart conditions. These groups of parents offer support and share their experience and hope. Take these or leave them but if you are so inclined a few suggestions include Fontan Rockstars, Heartmums, HRHS, HLHS, CHD support, Tricuspid Atresia Support Group and Heartkids Parents. Prenatal exercise classes and yoga are other ways of meeting expectant mums and sharing your experience.

If you are finding it hard to communicate your honest fears and worries with your partner, seek out an alternate support person you can confide in, perhaps your mum (biological or stand in), sister, close friend, someone you can really be honest with. There is a long road ahead but this is not impossible.

2.

20 WEEKS TO GO

Your baby may be categorised as a "high-risk pregnancy" following the diagnosis of their heart defect. Special care and a watchful eye is required to track the remaining weeks of your pregnancy. Sleep, exercise and your mental health should be high on your list of priorities.

The third trimester doesn't officially commence until the seventh month (or week 27) and will end on the day of induction/birth. Most pregnancies requiring Fontan Surgery will be induced to enable the best possible preparation for the first surgery and the organisation of the medical team.

You may find the third trimester more emotionally confronting as you prepare for the birth of your baby and the challenges to come. Try not to get lost in the worries, fears and "what if's" of this pregnancy. Your baby's heart condition is well and truly out of your control. It's important that you try to keep yourself comfortable and calm. You may like to consider self-care activities such as yoga or hydrotherapy.

During this period, your baby will continue to grow and you will likely gain more weight. You may want to consider buying or borrowing maternity clothing including comfortable maternity bras. Don't forget to consider breastfeeding options prior to buying maternity bras.

The final development of your baby's brain and lungs is also taking place during this time. You may notice "normal" pregnancy issues in your body like heartburn, leg cramps, back pain, difficulty sleeping, physical discomfort, and fatigue. Remember to consult with your midwife or cardiologist before using any new medications, natural supplements, remedies, or other alternative treatments.

This period may also be the time when you're preparing a nursery and buying all the necessary equipment and clothing for your newborn. Some of the items you require may include:

- **Baby clothes** – any clothing items that can accommodate wires, tubes and hospital cords should be considered. However, keep in mind that the hospital usually provides the required clothing whilst your baby is in their care. A bare baby provides easier observations for the teams of people who will rotate around your baby's bedside. Some specialty baby clothing manufacturers make clothing items for hospital bubs. Check out this possibility online if you have the time and feel the need.

- **Baby monitor** – it's wise to discuss this item with your doctor as some brands have video and audio features and some can track breathing, heart rate, etc. Please consider whether this item may cause more stress than relief if you're likely to over-focus on the monitor and sleeping baby.

- **Pram** – if (like me) you were given no guarantee that your baby would survive the pregnancy, birth or early surgery, you may want to consider whether you prefer to delay buying expensive items. I decided to buy only essential items for my newborn to avoid having to dispose of them if my baby didn't survive. It's not a pleasant thought and not one I dwelled upon, yet one that you need to take into account as part of your planning.

This period before birthing also provides time to revisit your self-care options, add as many to your list as possible while you can. The road ahead can be exhausting and sleep may be hard to come by as hospitals are busy and noisy places. You might consider prenatal massage, floatation or a hydrotherapy class for pregnant mums. You may also wish to consider seeing a psychologist or counsellor to talk through your fears and experiences and to identify self-care and coping strategies. Your pregnancy is one part of this CHD journey and there is a precious birth, followed by a minimum of three surgeries before your baby receives a fully functional Fontan circulation.

This journey will be challenging and scary at times. At a minimum, you are likely to have three experiences of handing your baby over to a stranger in a sterile operating theatre for life-saving surgery. The more support you can engage, the more coping strategies you have access to from the outset, the better prepared you may find yourself and therefore the better you will be able to manage future situations.

You may have to travel long distances to the hospital, depending on where your medical team plan to complete the induction and delivery of your baby. Someone within the midwifery team of the designated hospital will now become part of your team and a very important organiser. Regular, future appointments will be scheduled with that person. Further scans of your baby will also be organised. Together, all the people in your team will keep a close eye on the development of your baby and of course, you.

You will also have separate future visits (usually coordinated during the same visit if travelling any distance) with your baby's cardiologist. He or she will conduct an echocardiograph (see glossary) on your baby's heart – this is similar to a regular ultrasound and is non-invasive.

I can only suggest that if you haven't already done so, grab yourself a diary as a means of getting yourself super organised. There will be lots

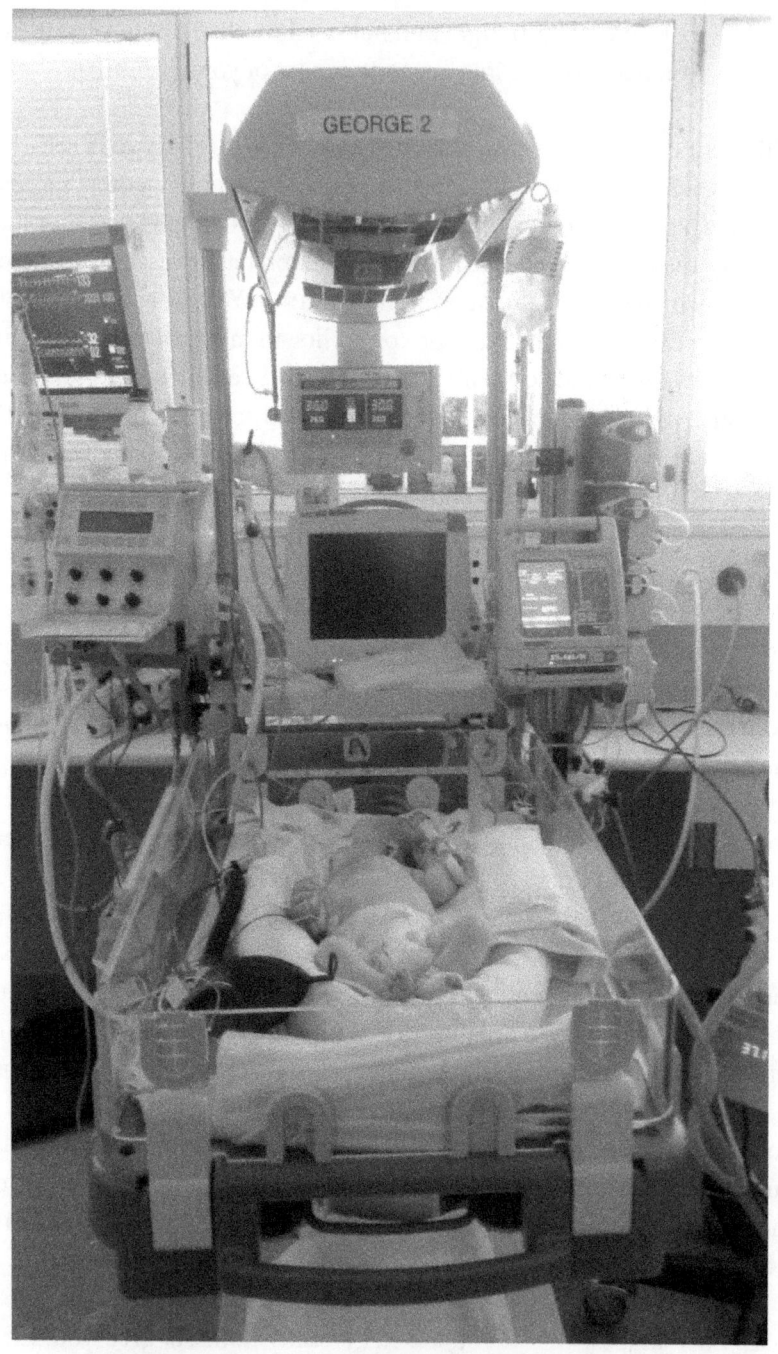

Daniel recovering on "George 2" after his 1st heart surgery

of medical appointments and data to record. A diary or folder will make it easier to record and find information when needed. Packing a water bottle and snacks to keep you nourished can make lengthy hospital visits easier to cope with.

Discuss your birthing options with your midwife or the doctor who will deliver your baby. Sometimes a natural birth is not possible due to the nature of the heart defect. Don't forget to discuss pain relief options. If you really want to avoid a caesarean birth, talk to your doctor. The hospital will provide you with all the information necessary for planning the best options for you and your baby.

Depending on the hospital, you may also be offered an orientation of the Neonatal Intensive Care Unit, commonly referred to as the NICU (this can be in a totally separate hospital depending on the set up of the birthing suite and the NICU). If you feel up to it and it hasn't been offered, ask for a tour to prepare yourself for your first visit there. Keep in mind this can be a confronting and emotional experience. Ask if there is an information pack and seek out any material that may make your arrival easier.

It may also be worth considering asking for a tour of the birthing unit and hospital if one is not offered to you. Become familiar with the room in which you may give birth and ask about options if these rooms are full on the day. Keep in mind that a team of medical staff will be present for the birth of your baby. These people will conduct the required duties and checks to transport your baby to the NICU as soon as possible following birth.

Please consider that you may or may not get to meet your baby before departure from the birthing room. Your baby may be taken away for immediate surgery or intervention before your first cuddle. This possibility can be discussed prior to the birth, but keep in mind that plans can and do change. Your baby's health and survival are the priority. Try not to worry, ask your partner or support person to accompany your baby to the NICU and stay bedside until you arrive. Consider whether you need an extra set of hands or another support person to remain with you while a midwife assists in the delivery of the placenta and finalises any caesarean arrangements.

Complications can occur during the birthing process at any time. It is highly likely that during labour you will be wearing a monitor around your baby bump. This belt will track baby's heart rate and vitals. If you were planning on a natural delivery and circumstances change during the birth, your birthing plan will need to change.

Post-birth, complications or delays may also arise and prevent you from physically arriving at the NICU as anticipated. No-one knows what lies ahead but don't be surprised if you find yourself in the Fontan Dance at this time. Hospitals have rules and procedures. You can't change or fight these in a matter of minutes, so weigh up what is most important and which battles you have to fight. When the time is right, you will get that first cuddle with your baby.

There is a lot of hospital equipment that will become familiar to you over the next few years (e.g. the monitoring devices and what they measure, the oxygen saturation monitors, etc.). One piece of confronting equipment that you may get to see and examine prior to your baby needing it, is what we in Australia call "George". This piece of equipment is also known as an "open care system". This large bed on wheels has many attachments including various monitors, recording devices, an overhead heater, suction, oxygen and so on. George is battery operated and includes the life-saving equipment sometimes required if your baby should need emergency treatment whilst in transit from one ward to another or to theatre. The actual item can be confronting. It is even more confronting when you see your baby for the first time surrounded by the swarm of professionals conducting their duties and checks. If possible, check George out before induction day. This apparatus is equally as amazing as the people trained to use and operate it.

Breastfeeding is worth discussing with your midwife or doctor prior to the arrival of your baby. Is it likely to be possible? Are you planning on breastfeeding? What is your preference? Breastfeeding your baby is a personal choice and sometimes not possible with a special care baby. Talk to your midwife or doctor about options.

The majority of babies in the NICU will be tube fed. A nasal gastric tube (NG) may have been inserted into your baby's body and will be taped to the side of their cheek and inserted up a nostril. There is no pain associated with the NG tube for your baby. It is designed to provide precious fluid for hydration and comfort. This is a bidirectional, flexible, rubber or plastic tube passed through the nose, down through the nasopharynx and oesophagus into the stomach.

Be prepared that on the first visit to your baby, he or she may have the NG tube (and other attachments) already inserted. You may have seen a baby with an NG tube during your hospital orientation. Such an experience is worthwhile in preparing yourself for this first meeting. It is an emotional time and you may be feeling overwhelmed and exhausted post-birth. Expect to see the NG tube. Remember the staff in the NICU will take good care of your baby while you try to get some rest.

Depending on your hospital, you may be encouraged to express prenatal colostrum for your baby's first feeds (sometimes referred to as harvesting). There's an art to getting the hang of massaging your nipple to express one drop of colostrum at a time. Talk to your midwife and seek out the time when you should commence expressing and storage. Colostrum is frozen and stored in syringes within the hospital system. Follow the instructions provided and carefully label and store your stock.

Some professionals will say it is simply not possible to breastfeed your baby given the amount of energy required by the newborn. It might be a possibility but it can be exhausting for baby as they get closer to heart failure. Storing your breastmilk and freezing it is a great option for baby.

Babies born with CHD are highly likely to reach the point of heart failure before Fontan Surgery. Take a breath and pause here – heart failure does

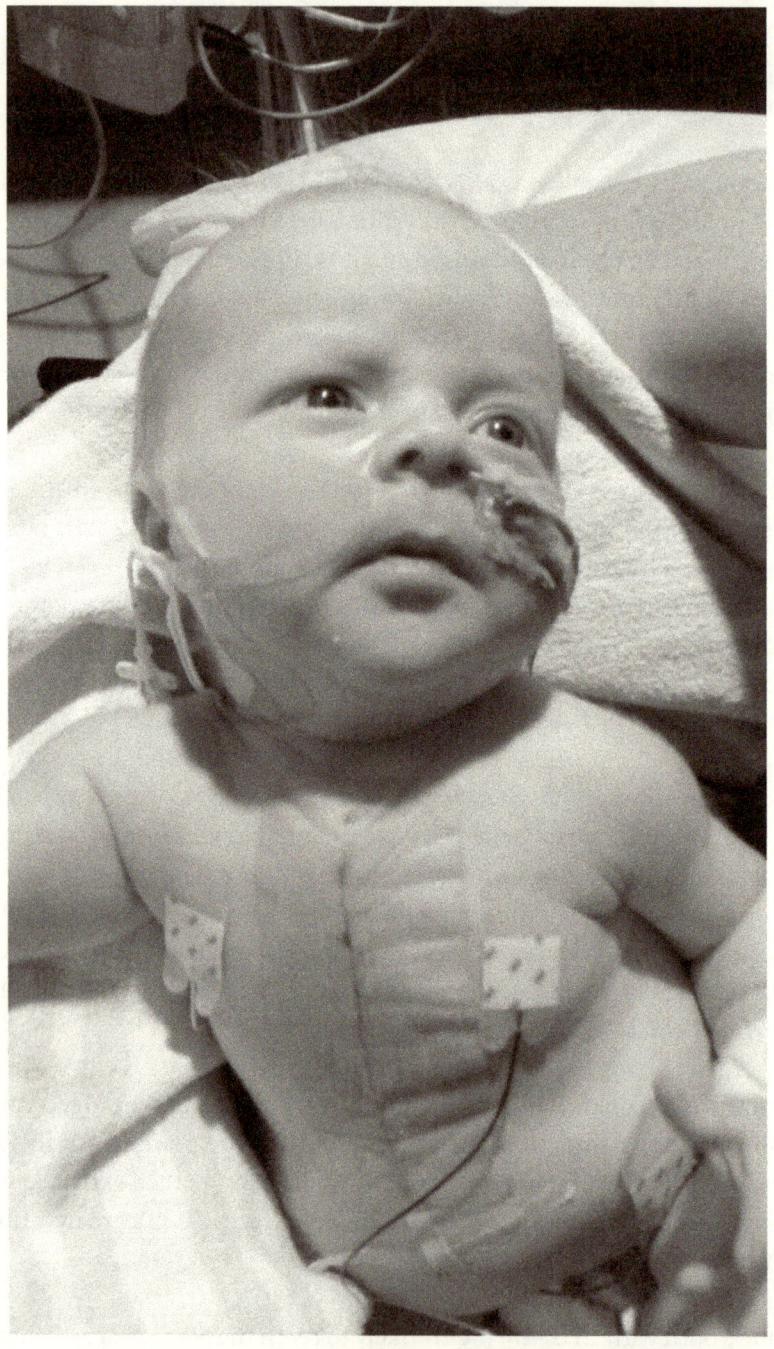

See nasal gastric tube plus monitoring leads and new zipper

not mean that your child is dying. Your baby can remain in the state of heart failure for weeks, months and even years depending on how they cope with the effects of failure and the plan for surgery. Symptoms of heart failure can include, but are not limited to: rapid breathing or shortness of breath, fatigue, falling asleep or becoming too tired to get through a breastfeed, lack of appetite, poor weight gain, an increase in sweating and more.

Symptoms of CHD may present as a bluish or purple tint to the skin (particularly around the nose and mouth area) and bluish fingernails and lips. This is called cyanosis, which is basically a lack of oxygenated blood (you will get very used to these symptoms).

Blaming yourself? It is highly likely that nothing and no-one is to blame for this malformation in your baby's heart. However, many mothers blame themselves and wonder what they did wrong at what stage in the early weeks of pregnancy. It's a tough pill to swallow but you will eventually get used to it. There is nothing you can do to reverse the condition. This is fate, maybe you want to call it bad luck? Statistics tell us that one in eight babies in Australia every day is born with a CHD and these figures are on the rise. So whatever you think you may have done or refrained from doing, remember that 85–90% of heart defects have no known cause or origin. You are not to blame.

One positive at this stage is that if you already have sought out this handbook, it is highly likely that your baby's defect has been detected while in utero. This is a strong place to be in for getting yourself organised and mentally prepared for the remainder of the pregnancy, the birthing experience, and the surgical pathway that lies ahead. Some mums don't have the luxury of having the defect detected prior to birth and are thrown in the deep end of CHD on the day their baby arrives or shortly after arriving home. Make sure that you make use of any time you have as best you can. Each step along the way will provide you with amazing and rewarding experiences. The choices ahead are totally yours and the words within these following chapters are put forward as shared information that I hope will be helpful rather than confronting.

You may wish to research grief or talk about it with a therapist. Talking about your own grief experience with someone you trust can be invaluable before induction day to help process any feelings you are experiencing. A written diary can assist in this process too. Most mums will experience some form of grief along this journey, it may come and go and this is natural, there are many things to grieve. Don't forget that your attitude can and will have a bearing on this journey ahead. Keep an open mind and try to remain as positive as you can. There is a large community of support and encouragement available along this journey.

Your accommodation options (and perhaps information for family and or friends who may like to visit you) are also something worth researching at this point. Some hospitals will have limited internal accommodation available close to the NICU. Ask your midwife, social worker or ward clerk for a list of accommodation options to consider. Familiarise yourself with the options and places you know you may be staying prior to your arrival to ensure you are organised. Also put these same details into the folder you started. You might also consider checking the hospital website, as they may have information available with contact details for accommodation options, maps, prices, etc.

3.

THE F WORDS

I AM NOT GOING to start this chapter with the four letter F word that we all know very well and may have been repeating religiously since diagnosis. However, if that word provides you with some relief, go on and say it as loud and as often as you like as there is real power in the spoken and screamed word. The following other F words will hopefully provide you with some ideas to consider as you progress through this precious pregnancy.

#1. Fontan

Doctor Francis Fontan was the mastermind and legend behind the life-saving surgery that your baby will undergo in the near future. The surgery is usually conducted in three stages, all performed at various periods of life depending on the condition and progress.

Francis Fontan, born in Nay, France (1929–2017), trained in cardiology and surgery at the University of Bordeaux to become one of the world's most highly recognised and respected surgeons in the cardiac field, particularly CHD.

On the 25th April 1968, Doctor Fontan and his colleague Eugene Baudet conducted the first Fontan procedure on a 12-year-old French girl with Tricuspid Atresia. She survived the surgery. Doctor Fontan connected her inferior vena cava, carrying the deoxygenated blood from her body, directly to her pulmonary artery and into her lungs. In 1970, Doctor Fontan did a similar successful procedure on another patient with Tricuspid Atresia, this time with fewer postoperative complications. The cardiac world learned of this surgical success in 1971 when the results of these surgeries were first published.

The Fontan procedure is now known and used worldwide. Doctor Fontan was active in many types of CHD surgery and was a pioneer of heart transplantation in France. The Fontan procedure (already modified three times over the past 50 years) refers to any heart surgery that results in the flow of systemic venous blood to the lungs without passing through a ventricle. It is a palliative surgical option, and is used to treat several complex congenital heart abnormalities.

Between 1968 and 1990, the Atriopulmonary Fontan Procedure, Doctor Fontan's first version, was the form most commonly used by surgeons worldwide. This was then modified, improved and superseded by the Lateral Tunnel Fontan Procedure, which remained in place until the turn of the century. With advances in technology and material, the Extracardiac Conduit Procedure is now the most current, popular and successful version.

The Extracardiac Conduit version sees the superior vena cava connected to the right pulmonary artery. The inferior vena cava is then re-routed through a Gore-Tex tube (sometimes called a conduit), which runs outside the heart and is connected to the pulmonary arteries. During this surgery the atrial septum is removed (usually in a previous surgery at an earlier stage). Blood returns via the pulmonary veins into the left atrium and may also pass to the right atrium freely.

3 TYPES OF FONTAN

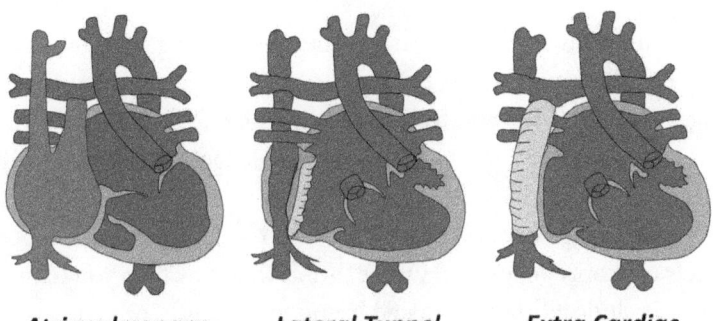

Atriopulmonary   *Lateral Tunnel*   *Extra Cardiac*

Without the courage, brilliance and curious mind of Francis Fontan, thousands of patients worldwide would not be able to receive this life-saving surgery every year. May he rest in peace and be satisfied that his technique and curiosity has saved the lives of countless babies.

Latter chapters in this book will outline each of the three stages of the Extracardiac Conduit Version of Fontan Surgery (which is the only experience that I can share with you). Stage one, usually performed at birth or shortly afterwards, consists of the pulmonary artery banding or sometimes a shunt (depending on the nature of your baby's problem). Stage two is usually performed around six months of age and is called the Bidirectional Glenn Shunt. The third open heart surgery sees the final connection of a new circulation called Fontan (the timing of this surgery can vary significantly depending on progress).

#2. Fear

CHD is a new and scary place to be. It can present you with a new type of fear, which may be glaringly obvious. My fear was not so much in the birthing stage of this pregnancy, but was instead the constant fear in the lead up to his birth day of, "Is he going to be ok?" "Is he going to survive?"

"Will he be blue?" "How will I cope?" "What might happen?" There are plenty of unknowns and a total lack of control.

What is fear? Fear is a challenging emotion often triggered by an actual or perceived threat of danger, pain, or harm. Fear is a natural and normal feeling – it is good for you to be aware of the effect that fear is having within your body. It is okay to notice, acknowledge and try to deal with it.

How can you survive this fear? One idea is to seek professional support if that feels appropriate for you. Other things that may help you to manage your fear include talking to trusted friends and family, or giving yourself permission to be scared, to cry, and to feel your pain and fear. Journalling or writing a diary can offer you a place to scribble out your worries and thoughts without having to deal with anyone else's reaction or judgements.

I have often read back through my diary of those early days after diagnosis to find the strength and courage, to see the big picture and work through conquering my fear.

Depending on how you are coping with the news of the recent diagnosis and how comfortable you feel in communicating this with your loved ones, potentially young children, family members and friends, it might be time to think about the best method of disclosing your baby's diagnosis. This can be a challenge and upsetting for you as well as the person you are sharing the news with. Take your time – explaining a condition that is foreign to you can be challenging, and it's normal to feel emotional when talking about this. It is not a straightforward explanation to try to explain or repeat to loved ones. Another option to consider is to hand them a fact sheet from the hospital or printed off the hospital website on Fontan Surgery.

Given you are obviously pregnant and your baby bump continues to expand, it is normal for even "Joe Public" to comment on your bump, ask you questions about when your due date is, whether you know the sex of your baby and even (God forbid) those random members of the public who feel they have the right and urge to touch your bump or body (be prepared). You don't have to tell anyone your news or your fears of your baby's diagnosis. You have the right to put your own needs first and manage your priorities.

In my experience, I told people the minimum as it was something I found difficult and awkward. Think it over and be prepared to respond in ways that may surprise or upset you for no apparent reason. People often mean well but don't know what to say. They can and will make stupid comments that are hard to forget. Have a think about the need to explain a potentially long absence and birthing experience to the school for your older children when you are ready.

#3. Faith: What exactly is it?

Faith is a personal thing. For me, it simply means believing that something is true and then committing my life to it and its practices. Some humans are born into a faith and grow up surrounded by certain practices and beliefs, others can discover faith later in life. Faith can simply refer to a trust or confidence, an assurance, or any belief.

For those mums with faith, a small item to keep in your pocket or handbag on stressful days can be handy. Pack this in your hospital bag – things such as medals, mala beads, rosary beads, holy cards, relics or other precious items that were gifted or bought for you or your baby. Your faith and any reminder of your own God's love will be required every step of the way to Fontan surgery and beyond.

For those other mums without faith, there are plenty of options available for you too, including quiet rooms within the hospital in case you need to snatch a period of time to meditate, chill out and do whatever it is that you do best and that helps to cope.

The expression "just have faith, it will work out" is used by some people to encourage and comfort anyone facing a serious problem, or in our case, a recent diagnosis of a potentially life-threatening CHD. In my experience, faith and prayer to any Higher Power can make us all feel calm and loved. You may find yourself feeling supported by family, your congregation, a support group, and the people you are about to meet along this journey. For me, knowing that people were praying for me and my baby also provided comfort.

Many priests and ministers of various faiths will grant a special blessing to any person who seeks it. If you are considering the people and F's to enlist on your team in preparation for Fontan, please don't dismiss the strength that you may gain from believing in a Higher Power and by asking for guidance and help to get through the journey ahead. The majority of major hospitals provide a chapel or quiet room for prayer, meditations and reflection.

Alternatives to the #3 F may include meditation, prayer and mindfulness. There are lots and lots of courses available, some are free, others are not (many are available online). Don't underestimate the strength you may get from engaging in your faith or finding a new one. Challenging times lie ahead.

#4. Family and Friends

Enlisting the support and help from the precious people within your network will be invaluable. Don't be afraid to ask for help (even if you are not usually so inclined). People will want to be able to do something practical to assist you on this journey so farm out the jobs that can be farmed out and take some of the load off your shoulders. Some suggestions might be to ask for frozen meals to stock up your freezer, assistance with transport of siblings to and from school or extra curricula activities, help with housework, lawn mowing, shopping for baby items, or just time for a cup of tea and a chat.

Look at your list of "things to do" and delegate some of those mundane or harder to deal with items. At times throughout this journey you may find yourself away from the family home for weeks, even months, depending on progress. Frozen meals are a godsend. Don't be shy to share your favourite menu either, as this can make life easier for those trying to be supportive by providing a meal for your children that they will actually eat.

One suggestion to help family and friends who may be holding the fort while you're in hospital or interstate is to compile a booklet of useful information. My booklet included emergency numbers of friends and family who were part of our network, a simple routine written out describing what duties were required from Monday to Sunday, which child needed to be where, which bin was supposed to be in the front driveway, when any deliveries might be expected, and so on. I also included teachers' names and phone numbers, and the email addresses of teaching staff and front office personnel.

#5. Facebook

Facebook is a communication tool available for you to utilise or consider establishing if you are not already a "user" or don't have an account. A closed or private group can be a great idea and opportunity to communicate with a group of people when time is precious. You can include only the people you want to share your journey with, and you can add photos and updates accordingly. The posts can later provide a precious document or diary of all that you communicated with those close to you.

4.

THE VARIETY OF HOSPITAL STAYS AND VISITS

For the next few years you may find yourself coming and going from the childrens' hospital. In the early years of your baby's life, it will be busy – expect that. It's common to undergo the first two stages of heart surgery in the lead up to your baby's Fontan and highly likely that this may happen in the first twelve months of their life. There may or may not be additional short and long hospitalisations depending on your baby's health.

Some babies will be able to go home shortly after birth, some may not leave hospital for weeks or months, and sadly, some will die. In Australia, CHD is the leading cause of infant death under the age of one, with four infant deaths per week (2020 Statistics). These are the cruel facts of the "team" you never wanted to join. The good news is that you've joined a team of people who appreciate life in a delightful way. "Heartkids", "Heartmums" and their families generally have a zest for life and health once the surgeries and hospital stays are over for the majority and your "new normal" kicks in.

You probably have some kind of plan for your baby's birth and early life. You need to be aware that this plan can change in unexpected and unwanted ways. For example, you may find yourself remaining in hospital for weeks or even months. I suggest that you make a plan with your cardiology team and midwives, ask questions, consider their advice, and also pay attention to your motherly instinct. If something doesn't feel right, advocate and ask questions until you are satisfied you have enough information.

This chapter offers some suggestions for your hospital visits: what to consider packing for yourself and your baby, what you might need when leaving hospital, return visits and longer stays.

Packing the hospital bag

First, you need to consider the possibility that you may have a lengthy stay in hospital after the birth and will therefore need to pack more items. My suggestion is that you pack a separate bag for each family member. Separating your items from your baby's items will make it quicker and easier to find what you need. It may be useful to pack a separate bag for your partner too. This way items are not taken home, lost between bags, or difficult or time-consuming to find. Anything you can do to relieve stress when you are exhausted and sleep deprived is worth considering.

For Mum

Toiletries: shampoo and conditioner, body wash or soap, brush/comb, hairdryer, moisturiser, hand cream, chap stick or lip balm (lips can get dry in the air conditioning for long periods), razor, deodorant, toothbrush and toothpaste, perfume, hairbands, paracetamol, any other prescription medications, eye mask (to block the light when trying to sleep), earplugs, a small torch and spare torch battery (to aid you in the middle of the night), oils (lavender drops on the pillow might help you sleep), any other aide or item that can assist you to relax and get some rest/sleep (massage oil, diffuser, etc.).

Other items: mobile phone and charger, iPad (tablet, laptop, kindle) or any device to keep you busy/distracted and its charger, books to read, a writing pad and pen, a journal for baby, pencils and highlighter, laundry detergent, a small bag with coins (for vending machines or coin operated laundry machines), a towel, pillow case and even a face washer from home (preferably one that smells like home), umbrella, alarm clock, extension cord, power board, sports water bottle and snacks.

Clothes: underpants, bras, socks, a warm jumper or two, comfortable pants (e.g. yoga or tracksuit), pyjamas, shirts and loose fitting tops, a scarf to keep you warm, a hat if you get to go outside, thongs (for shower), comfortable shoes and/or slippers.

Maternity items: nursing bras, breast pads, sanitary pads, breastfeeding equipment (bottles, teats, sterilisers, formula powder, cleaning agents), breast pump, creams for post birth and anything else you can think of.

For Baby

The hospital will usually provide every item required from baby's first dummy (expect your baby to be sucking this when you first meet him or her), beanie/bonnet to keep the head warm, small clothing gowns and suits (depending on wiring and leads attached to baby), to nappies, creams, bath wash, etc.

Remember to clearly label any items you bring from home with your name and keep an eye on them as they can end up in the hospital laundry and be lost forever (or stolen as thieves also visit all sections of the hospital).

It can be nice to bring along some of your own items from home such as baby wraps to swaddle, suits, a small teddy bear or a soft toy to remain in the crib with baby, socks, a knitted hat/beanie, some toys that can distract baby, books, your own music and lullabies, clothes to travel home in, and don't forget the baby capsule or you won't actually be leaving hospital! The capsule should have previously been fitted to your vehicle and checked for safety – add this item to your to do list.

Every hospital is different but most provide similar facilities for families. Vending machines on the wards provide you with access to drinks and snack foods and sometimes even a variety of frozen meals which can be microwaved in parent facilities/tea rooms. Check out the website of the hospital and see what's offered and where things are located. Become especially familiar with car parking arrangements for long-term stays and the cost. Anything else you can bring from home in preparation for a long stay will save you time and stress when you're exhausted. Check out the cafes and cafeteria options as well as the location of the coffee cart or shop.

Some hospitals provide parent accommodation located close to the NICU. Try to visit this facility if you can. Consider what facilities you might use and make a booking if it is an option. Inspect the kitchen and bathroom and ask to see an empty room. They usually offer a small bed and limited furniture. Even though this accommodation can be very basic, if it's close to the NICU and your baby, it's a godsend. Research other accommodation options off hospital campus and ask for a hospital rate if you are staying long term as many places provide a discounted rate. Consider your budget and of course the distance from the hospital. The NICU will have your contact number while your baby remains there and they will call you if you're required to return to your baby.

Consider taking some personal items to remind you of home: a small photo book of a recent holiday, photos of your other children and family, your favourite family photo, drawings from older siblings to add some colour and love into your temporary bedroom, blue tac or sticky tape to attach them to walls or the back of a door, something warm that smells like home (a small blanket, scarf or favourite top), scribbling pads, colouring in and crossword books (or any other item that may help you pass the time while you sit bedside with your baby), a pillow and pillowcase from home or something small to add extra comfort.

The birth

It's a huge day in this journey and a massive event in your life. It's equally as exciting as it is terrifying. If you've done your preparation there's nothing more for you to do right now.

If you feel like you need an early meditation or prayer before heading into the hospital, there are plenty of free options available via apps on your phone if you don't have an off the cuff favourite. Alternatively, there's usually a quiet room or chapel within the hospital grounds.

You might be feeling a mix of excitement and fear at this point but if possible, try to eat a decent breakfast before heading into the hospital. A good breakfast (if you can manage to eat) will provide you with some energy stores that will be required for today and beyond. Remember to keep hydrated throughout the morning and pack some high energy snacks or fruit in your bag too.

Arrive early, or at least on time, with all the goodies you will need or plan to use during the birth. Try to stay flexible and remember that labour can be unpredictable and may not be the same as previous birthing experiences. The ultimate goal on this day is to keep mum and baby healthy and get baby across to the NICU for appropriate care as soon as possible.

The hospital will have provided you with instructions for your induction or planned C-section. You should have already discussed pain-management options and written down your choices. Your birthing options may have also been documented (for example water therapy which might be out of the question if you are attached to monitoring equipment). Make sure you have discussed with your team any major queries or concerns prior to this day. If not, raise them now – forewarned is forearmed.

Your day may start in a separate area of the hospital as opposed to where you may finish up post-birth. The induction process could be performed in the day unit or another area. Usually, the doctor begins induction by checking your cervix and looking for signs of dilation. Most commonly, a prostaglandin gel is applied to gently encourage labour to begin. Alternatively, intravenous oxytocin may be used to start contractions (this speeds up labour and is administered via a drip which will restrict your movement).

During labour, staff will check your blood pressure and temperature. They may take blood or request a urine sample too. They may also strap a monitor to your belly to track baby's heart rate and the frequency of contractions. This precious data enables your team to best support your baby and helps them determine their surgery plan. Designated staff elsewhere in the childrens' hospital are possibly also awaiting the arrival of your precious baby. Lean on your partner or support person and do your best to labour through the contractions as they come and go.

If you are planning to be active throughout your labour you should discuss this with the midwife and ask about intermittent monitoring to allow you the freedom to move around. Keep in mind, you may be asked to stay in bed to allow monitoring – try to go with the flow and enjoy the experience if possible.

At some point, you'll be confined to the designated birthing room where you'll see the familiar medical trolley bed (that we call George) and a range of other equipment. When the baby's head crowns during a natural birth, additional professionals will likely enter your room (maybe 8–10 people). Try to ignore them, they'll keep quiet and out of the way while you deliver your precious baby.

The team will need to conduct checks of your baby immediately after birth. It's possible that you may have to wait for the first feed and cuddle with your new baby. Your support person will hopefully have the option to cut the umbilical cord and shortly after you may even catch a glimpse of your newborn baby, who might be quiet or crying loudly. Your baby is probably now lying on their back on the George mattress surrounded by the team. Try to relax for a moment and take in the realisation that your baby has finally been born. The midwife will assist in the delivery of the placenta and will provide you with any further self-care instructions.

Post-delivery

If the plan for your baby was immediate surgery after birth, arrangements will be made for you to arrive at the NICU or elsewhere as soon as practical. Remember that your baby is in good hands during this separation and right now you need to focus on your recovery from the birth. It's important to note that your delivery may not have gone to plan. Unexpected complications including the incomplete delivery of the placenta, haemorrhage, blood clot, infection, chest pain, etc. can occur. Listen to the midwife and follow the instructions given to you.

If your baby is undergoing surgery, you may be afforded a short rest now. Otherwise, you may be taken to the NICU via wheelchair for your first visit with your new baby. Remember to save your energy and take your recovery gently. This first meeting is emotional, so try to prepare yourself. Hopefully you have been advised as to what condition your baby is in – NG tube, a breathing machine, monitoring, etc. If there's a multitude of connections assisting your baby, you may not be able to pick him or her up. It may feel like there's barely any skin visible between the cords, wires, tubes and monitors supporting your baby. It can be distressing to see your new baby with a range of foreign attachments, but these devices are supporting your precious baby.

The NICU can be noisy and there can be an unexpected emergency being attended to. Take your arrival gently and move slowly. Enjoy your first meeting and follow the advice and instructions of your midwife.

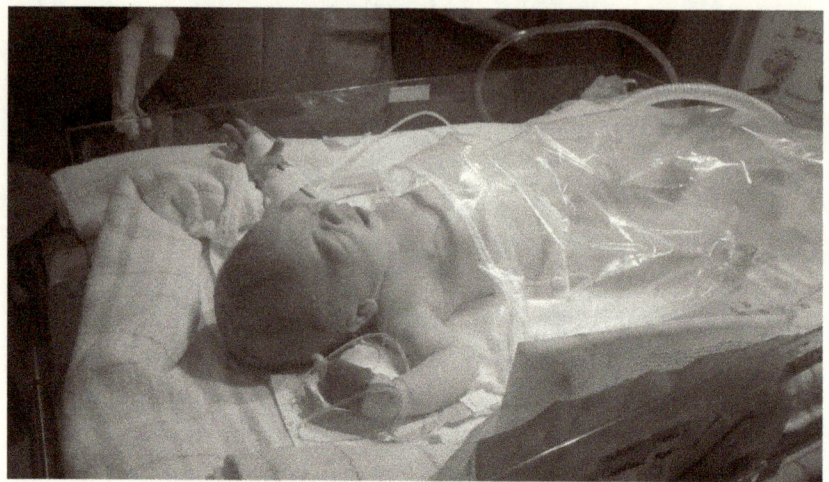
The first photo taken of Daniel whilst on "George 2"

Some tips for visiting the NICU:

- always wash your hands on entry and exit to the area
- follow the signs and instructions within your hospital
- try to leave any expensive items and other valuables at home
- there's usually a limit to the amount of visitors allowed in the NICU at one time and some hospitals have visiting hours (but generally parents are exempt)
- follow the guidelines regarding bringing food and hot drinks into this area.

Another experience that you may prefer to read about prior to being thrown in the deep end is when and if the power fails. This can and does happen in the main hospital and the NICU too. The high-risk babies are usually in a bed with ventilators and there are systems in place to keep your baby safe in this event. An emergency plan will be activated and the trained nurses will be moving gently but in full flight. Follow instructions provided by staff and do as you are told.

The NICU specialises in caring for babies with complex medical conditions, not only cardiac babies, though these occupy a large portion of the available

THE VARIETY OF HOSPITAL STAYS AND VISITS

beds. The neonatal period is defined as the first 28 days of life and most babies in the NICU are of this age, depending on bed availability and hospital issues. Some NICU beds are different to others and will have additional equipment nearby. Some hospitals separate the ventilator beds from the high dependency beds to make access to medical equipment easier for staff. There will often be a high care area within the NICU. You will likely see babies and their families come and go – the length of hospital stays vary and there will be a constant rotation of nurses, doctors, lactation specialists, occupational therapists, researchers, etc.

If you have brought in personal items from home to decorate your baby's area, you'll need to check with the nurse due to hygiene restrictions. Singing and reading to your baby is a great way to bond during this time in the NICU (even if you can't touch or hold your baby yet, they can still hear and recognise your voice). Don't hold back as this is a great time to strengthen your bond with your new baby.

If friends or family members offer to help, consider saying yes. Helpful things you could ask for might include cooking a meal, taking home your washing and returning it clean, helping out with older siblings, or sitting with your baby in the NICU while you take a short break or a power nap in the middle of the day (because day and night sometimes don't exist for a while). Don't be shy, there's a long and exhausting road ahead of you.

A baby diary can be a good way to pass hours in the NICU. Whether you prefer scrapbooking or simply recording your baby's milestones, this will be a precious record for yourself and your baby. Keeping a record of your time in the NICU and special occasions such as your first cuddle, baby's first smile or first bath can help to restore a sense of normality. You might even like to collect and stick items discarded from hospital into the diary like ECG print outs, leads from their monitoring, dots from their chest (as they are replaced) etc. Don't forget to record their progress, their medications, who was looking after them and any significant events.

Below is a list of the main staff working in the NICU. The sight of the teams of people assisting your baby can be overwhelming when you first arrive but you'll get used to them. These teams can include but are not limited to:

- The Consultants are the most senior medical professionals on the ward. These include:
  - Cardiology (medical) Consultants
  - Cardiothoracic Surgeon
  - Neonatologists
  - Intensivists.
- The Fellow (in training to be a specialist)
- Registrar (still in training and usually rotating through various wards within the hospital)
- Resident Doctors (usually 12–24 months out of medical school)
- The nurses:
  - Nurse Practitioners (usually a PhD in cardiology or extra training and can order tests, insert cannulas, etc.)
  - Cardiac Nurse Consultants
  - Nurse Managers
  - Nurse Unit Manager (NUM)
  - Access Nurses (the senior nurses in the area)
  - Team Leader
  - Regular Nurses.

The "pumping room"

Most hospitals have a designated area for breastfeeding mothers to express milk, usually open 24/7 except for daily cleaning. If your baby is being tube-fed you'll have the option of formula milk or breastmilk. If expressing, you may have to visit this room every 3–4 hours depending on your milk supply. You will be provided with instructions on how to store and label your milk, which is usually taken straight to the "storage room" where the milk can be frozen or stored in refrigerators. The nurses have access to the milk and are able to feed your baby overnight or if you are unavailable for any reason.

A few things to note: this room is very quiet, dimly lit and provides a great escape from the noisy ward. Be prepared to meet other mums who might be enjoying a break, expressing milk, or expressing emotions. These mums are here for a reason too and may be having a hard time.

It can be very handy to have your own expressing equipment as it enables you to express in your room, freeing you from needing to be in the NICU. You may find that a feeding routine supports you to take self-care breaks away from the bedside. Your sleep and recovery are important, especially if you are here alone. A midwife will monitor your post-birth recovery and milk capacity, especially in the early days when the milk comes in (usually around day three).

Discharge from the NICU

Some hospitals will move you into another area of the NICU and allow you time to "practice" taking your baby home before the event. This is called "rooming in" and can be nerve-racking initially but it is all good practice, especially given the nurses and doctors are within walking distance.

It may also be suggested that you practice placing your baby in the capsule and allowing him/her to rest or sleep whilst monitoring their oxygen levels and any changes prior to the first car ride home (especially if it is for a lengthy ride interstate). Having time to practice things like managing feeding tubes and administering daily medications can be confidence building. You're likely to have mixed emotions when you take your precious heartkid home so make the most of this experience if it is afforded to you (as some hospitals may be too busy to offer it). Be confident, master the new skills you need to know, and take the journey one step at a time.

You may want to consider a diary for keeping track of medication dosages, administration details, feed times, milk quantities, toileting habits, sleep habits, and any other relevant data that makes tracking progress and developmental milestones clear. The information can be handy when communicating any concerns or changes to your medical team.

Coming home with baby

You're almost set for discharge when you've passed the "rooming in" phase with the hospital team and you feel confident to manage your baby's care at home. You may have to collect medications from the pharmacy, which can take short or long periods of time depending on staffing, your order and hospital stock. Make sure you check the medications and labels, including the doses, and check that you have enough syringes or other equipment to get you off to a good start once you arrive home.

Packing up your accommodation space will also require consideration and planning. Leaving the NICU with your baby for the first time is very exciting and the last thing you need is to be weighed down with bags and equipment. Remember to take it slowly as hormones and emotions can sneak up on you without warning. It's a massive accomplishment to finally be leaving the hospital with your baby for the first time. Congratulations.

You will most likely need a referral to a paediatrician before discharge. A paediatrician can be a handy "go between" for checks between scheduled cardiology appointments. This professional may or may not be needed depending on the severity of your baby's condition and the distance you reside from the hospital. If you do require a paediatrician make sure you add their contact details into the folder with important information that's easy to access. You may have permission to phone or email your paaediatrician, cardiologist or nurse consultant, especially soon after discharge when you may have lots of questions, concerns and new experiences at home. Trust your gut and if something doesn't feel right, make the call or attend the nearest hospital.

It will be important for you to keep an eye on the blueness or skin colour of your baby, which provides an indicator of their oxygen levels. Each baby will be different but most heart kids have decreased oxygen levels. Some

THE VARIETY OF HOSPITAL STAYS AND VISITS

parents might opt for a home-based moniroting device, others might attend the local hospital or rely on their paediatrician. Oxygen levels vary depending on your baby's Fontan stage, their overall health, and their level of activity. Your doctor will discuss this with you.

You will become a master at medication administration which will also vary before and after your baby's Fontan, e.g. diuretics are a common medication to keep fluids away from the organs in heart-babies. Your doctor will explain the medications your baby has been prescribed. Some babies will also be prescribed post-op Warfarin, others will be given daily Aspro – these medications help to keep the blood thin to reduce clotting.

You may like to consider writing a list of minimum required items should you unexpectedly need to attend hospital. Many heart-babies have a compromised immune system and are prone to catching the odd virus or illness. Consider things such as your baby's health record, health care cards, letter from paediatrician/cardiologist outlining their condition, breast pump, dummy and medications. You can gather these together and be well organised for if and when this occasion ever arises. Make sure you stick this list of "items to pack for emergency" somewhere handy.

One item worth considering for your own home is hand sanitiser and household disinfectant. After spending days, weeks, months within the hospital walls you will have become accustomed to hand washing and strict hygiene. It is worthwhile to insist that every visitor maintains this practice before entering your home. Make sure you check that visitors are healthy and unlikely to be carrying germs that could be spread to your baby. The last thing you need is additional time in hospital if it can be avoided.

Once you have settled into a routine at home you might like to connect with other heart mums via social media. It's ok if you want to focus on recovering from the hospital and birth and spending time with your baby, but these social media options can help with reducing feelings of isolation by providing a place to find support, new friends and shared hope. Many states and countries have their own heart parent community pages. You can contact HeartKids Australia and the ANZ Fontan Registry in Melbourne to find out more. Facebook community groups include the Fontan Rockstars, HLRH and HLHS, Heartkids Support, CHD awareness, Heartmums, and the Tricuspid Atresia Support Group. There are some wonderful groups and pages to help mums and adult heart kids who have lived experience of what you are going through.

Some parents may wish to consider setting up a medical alert item in their car to provide vital information for emergency service workers in the case of a motor vehicle accident. Think about how you can communicate your baby's heart condition to a stranger in an emergency. Perhaps consider attaching a laminated card to your baby's car seat. There are a multitude of medical alert bracelets, pouches for seatbelts etc. available online. These items may need to be updated as your child progresses through to Fontan stage and their needs change.

Patient travel scheme

Depending on where in the world you reside this scheme can be worth investigating. Some governments in some states (especially here in Australia) can offer financial assistance and rebates for interstate travel when your local hospital cannot provide the care required for your baby's heart condition. Check this scheme out with one of the nurse managers on the hospital ward, a social worker or better yet, another heart mum. If you meet the criteria, there can be financial assistance with fuel, transport and accommodation.

5.

HOSPITAL PROVISIONS

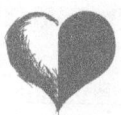

Babies admitted to the Neonatal Intensive Care Unit (NICU) are usually either premature or aged between birth and four weeks requiring intensive care. The specialist intensive care nurses in the NICU are trained to provide the highest level of medical attention and care to newborn babies.

In this unit, the staff congregate around the nursing station where they collect equipment and medications and conduct meetings. A ward clerk, often situated separately, is responsible for other important duties and can provide a wealth of information. Don't be shy in asking for advice or directions. If they can't advise you, they'll be able to refer you to someone who can.

The NICU will usually include one or two isolation rooms for babies who need to be separated. This may occur if a baby contracts a contagious virus, requires extra nursing, is receiving palliative care, or is experiencing other difficulties. The isolation rooms are quieter than the ward and you will need to follow the instructions and guidelines regarding hygiene protocols. Make sure you familiarise yourself with the emergency button in case your baby needs help and a nurse is not nearby.

There will usually be a tea room for parents in this area. Visiting hours and the number of people permitted into the unit at any one time are usually restricted.

The NICU will welcome you into a world that can be confronting, challenging and emotional. This unit cares for the sickest babies before they're discharged to another ward for continuing care. It's an extremely busy place and can be noisy with large groups of specialists meeting beside every baby, the constant beeping of the machinery and gentle chatter of staff and other families, not to mention the crying babies.

At one month of age, babies will usually be transferred from the NICU to the PICU (Paediatric Intensive Care Unit), which provides care for children aged between four weeks and 18 years of age. Generally, children are separated into age groups within the PICU when possible. The PICU will usually be larger than the NICU and can cater for more patients at one time.

Some hospitals may admit cardiac babies straight to the PICU (usually due to bed pressures).

You will often find small meeting rooms within these units where parents might meet with doctors following surgery, or they may be used as offices for various staff, medical supply rooms, equipment rooms, a kitchen for patients, a parent's tea room or lounge, a clothing store and so on. It's a good idea to walk around the unit when you need to stretch your legs and familiarise yourself with whose office is where and what services are provided. There is often a notice board for parents to keep up to date with hospital news, information and useful tips.

Separate to these two intensive care units, there's usually a specific cardiac ward for babies and children who require continuous but not intensive care. In here, the nurses deal solely with cardiac patients as opposed to the NICU and PICU nurses who care for young patients with a wide range of medical complaints. The ward and intensive care units each have a different feel, set-up and operation. The cardiac ward nurses are highly skilled in this one area, particularly post-Fontan surgery when the monitoring of fluids, drains and their output and removal are strictly monitored and removed at the correct time.

Many families will find the ward more relaxed, albeit extremely busy. Within the ward you will again see the isolation rooms made available when required. Some are single rooms whereas other rooms are larger and accommodate more children. The ward can be fun and a great place to make new friends and network with other heart families.

The ward will have a play room with toys and books for your child when he or she is well enough to get out of bed. There will be children of varying ages in this room so please be considerate of those children who are trying to sleep. You might like to ask if there are outdoor areas where your child can play in the fresh air and sunshine.

You will have access to a kitchen on the ward and over time you'll be able to be more active in your baby's care. Look for a fridge to store your grocery items. Some hospitals also have additional bed space on the ward for a parent to sneak in a nap (ask the nurse if one exists if it is not obvious to you).

Many specialists from other areas of the hospital visit the ward. The standard and rotating teams of medical professionals come and go daily, as do the research assistants and student doctors. Following Fontan surgery, blood samples are collected daily by the visiting phlebotomist (the technical name for the person drawing blood). Dieticians, physiotherapists, nurse educators, play therapists, music therapists, chaplains, social workers, volunteers and other people will also visit the ward. Try to take a break when you can. Wheelchairs and other mobility aides are available for you to take your child for a walk in the fresh air.

Try to maximise use of the options available to you. For example, you might check to see if there's a sibling care or day care option for your other children while you attend appointments. Most major hospitals will have a chemist, bank and various eating establishments as well as coffee bars. Speak to the parking office and see what type of permit you can purchase to reduce the costs of daily parking, particularly if you're staying for weeks. Word of mouth is a great way to learn about the services available to you. In saying that, it's normal to have times when you don't want to speak to anyone other than your child's team.

Most hospitals will have a library, hair salon and coin-operated laundry, and many will provide stalls where various groups hold fundraising events like cake and craft stalls.

Most will also have entertainment areas for the children where they can play games and watch movies, you may need to ask about wi-fi access. In-house, volunteers do a wonderful job of engaging children who are confined to the ward. Some hospitals will provide a room for siblings where they can access electronics, arts and crafts, musical instruments and so on. Keep your eyes and ears open for the range of opportunities available to keep your children happy and busy during the recovery period. The clown doctors are a real treat if they are available and active.

It can be handy to write down the operating hours of the cafeteria and other areas of the hospital you frequent. That way, if you know the cafeteria is closing at 9:00pm and you haven't eaten all day, you can get down there and get yourself a meal before it closes.

It's important to look after yourself, especially if you're alone caring for your baby. This can be a difficult, stressful, sleep deprived time. The nurses will record your phone number on the whiteboard beside the bed and will call you back in when needed. Try to have some faith in the people who are caring for your child, they are well trained and highly capable.

The quiet room can be a very busy place. Various denominations utilise this space and there will be a notice board advertising when different religions, services, prayer groups and Masses are held. A range of priests, ministers and representatives from a range of religions often share office space in this area of the hospital. You can write a request for prayers in the book.

A parent hostel is offered by some hospitals. The range of accommodation offered varies but is designed to meet the basic needs of parents caring for sick children. If available, the hostel will be situated close to the PICU and or NICU. Hostel space is limited and these rooms can fill up quickly. The rooms are small and basic, the bed will be small and probably uncomfortable, but it's good enough for a few hours rest in a location close to your baby. Have a look at the kitchen and bathroom in this area and ask the receptionist for an information pack.

6.

PULMONARY ARTERY BANDING OR SHUNT

SADLY, MANY PRECIOUS CHILDREN are born with various complex heart defects. These are known by various medical labels but you only need to focus on the name provided to you by your cardiologist. If your baby's heart defect qualifies for single ventricle surgery, they will usually require a three-staged surgical process. Fontan surgery is the third operation in this process.

The first process will usually include either a shunt or a band, which is inserted soon after birth. Your child's recovery will be unique but usually somewhere between 7–14 days. It is important to note that some babies, especially those born with defects like Hypoplastic Right Heart Syndrome (HRHS), require a major surgery involving the heart and lung machine in the days after birth, and will not have a shunt or a band. Nevertheless, the challenges arising can be similar in the post-operative period.

A shunt is made from a small tube of Gore-Tex (a similar material to what is used to make rain jackets). The tube is sewn to the blood vessels to increase blood flow to the lungs. This allows your baby's one heart ventricle to maintain sufficient blood oxygen levels.

The band is literally a small piece of material tied around the outside of the pulmonary artery. As the band is tightened, the artery narrows and blood flow is restricted which reduces the amount of blood going to the lungs to a level that the heart can manage, providing for both the lung and body circulations.

My aim in this chapter is to provide practical information to help prepare you for this procedure and hopefully reduce your fear of the unknown. Your baby will have one or the other, a band or a shunt in this first stage.

It is a hard task for any parent to hand a newborn baby over to a surgeon for heart surgery. The good news is that these surgeries are performed every day worldwide by experienced surgical teams. Try to have faith in the team, they are highly trained professionals, and follow the guidelines they provide to you.

The first stage is usually performed in the newborn period. Some babies will have this surgery very soon after birth, others may be may be able to wait a few weeks. Your cardiologist will discuss the surgical plan with you after he or she has performed that very first echocardiogram (known as an echo) on your baby's heart and completed an assessment of your baby's condition.

A few topics will come up in this chapter – the first of these is cyanosis.

Cyanosis is a blueish colour of the skin. This is usually seen around the face, fingers and toe nails. The colour can vary depending on physical movement and the heart's state of function. For example, crying may change your baby's colour, as can physical activity and current access to oxygen (e.g. sleep versus awake). The colour of cyanosis can vary from blue to purple and even shades of pink. Over time, you will become familiar with the changing colour of your baby's skin and their cyanosis.

PULMONARY ARTERY BANDING OR SHUNT

You will most likely notice cyanosis around the lips, nose or eyes of your baby. Their nail beds will appear purple too. You will discover that some people will notice the blue tinge and comment (sometimes rudely) whereas others will be oblivious. Just be aware that cyanosis and CHD go hand in hand with a single ventricle baby. Usually after Fontan surgery, the cyanosis will disappear or reduce significantly due to the new and improved circulation and increase in oxygen levels.

Heart failure is a stage that can last days, weeks, months, even years. It does not mean that death is imminent. Your baby may or may not go into heart failure. If they do, you are most likely to notice that they're sleeping more often and for longer periods of time, they'll appear different from normal, lethargic, easily fatigued from doing very little. While in heart failure, simple behaviours (like feeding) will reduce noticeably. Whereas before they would suck from the breast or bottle for 10 minutes, now they may only last 2–3 minutes and will likely fall asleep mid-suck.

It is a good idea to communicate any noticeable changes in your baby to your cardiologist. You might want to write them down with dates and times of your observations. Follow the instructions of your cardiologist. If you're worried, go to the nearest hospital.

Preparing for the first surgery will be different for each family and baby. Some babies will undergo the first stage soon after birth, other babies will be able to go home for a while before they enter heart failure. These babies will then return to hospital for their stage one surgery. If your baby is at home while you're anticipating heart failure, remember that good hygiene practices are critical for keeping your baby well. Viruses and infections can be easily contracted when the immune system is low.

It is natural for family and friends to want to visit but be mindful of the potential germs that every person entering your home is capable of sharing with baby.

Consider asking people to use face masks if they want to get close to your baby. Hand washing is essential before picking up your baby for a cuddle or assisting with bottle feeding, and with bathing and changing nappies. Many stores and pharmacy's stock antibacterial gel which can be carried with you at all times. Anything you can do to avoid bringing infection to your baby is worth considering.

You may want to restrict visitors until the first surgery has been completed, and you may consider putting signage up at the front door or entrance to remind people of hygiene instructions, especially if you feel awkward asking them to comply. I have seen some mothers put a sign on the pram asking people not to get too close or touch the baby. It is difficult to stop airborne germs and bugs, particularly in the hospital, but some measures can be put in place if you feel it is suitable for your circumstances.

Pre-admission stage

When the time is right, you will be required to attend hospital for stage one surgery. There is usually some form of pre-admission testing required a day or two before surgery and sometimes these tests are split over two days as they can be time-consuming. You will have been provided with instructions to follow. Be sure to call the hospital with any issues or questions you may have before arriving. Some of the preliminary tests might include:

- Measurements of baby's height, weight and head circumference
- An ECG will be conducted
- Bloods will be sent to pathology for testing before theatre
- Chest x-ray
- Echo.

Some hospitals will have mobile equipment (ECG, echo and even X-ray) which can be brought to the wards when required. Other hospitals will require that the patient be taken to special areas within the hospital to access the equipment. There can be long distances between wards so I suggest that you take a pram. Over time you will become familiar with the range of equipment required for your baby and which item is used for

PULMONARY ARTERY BANDING OR SHUNT

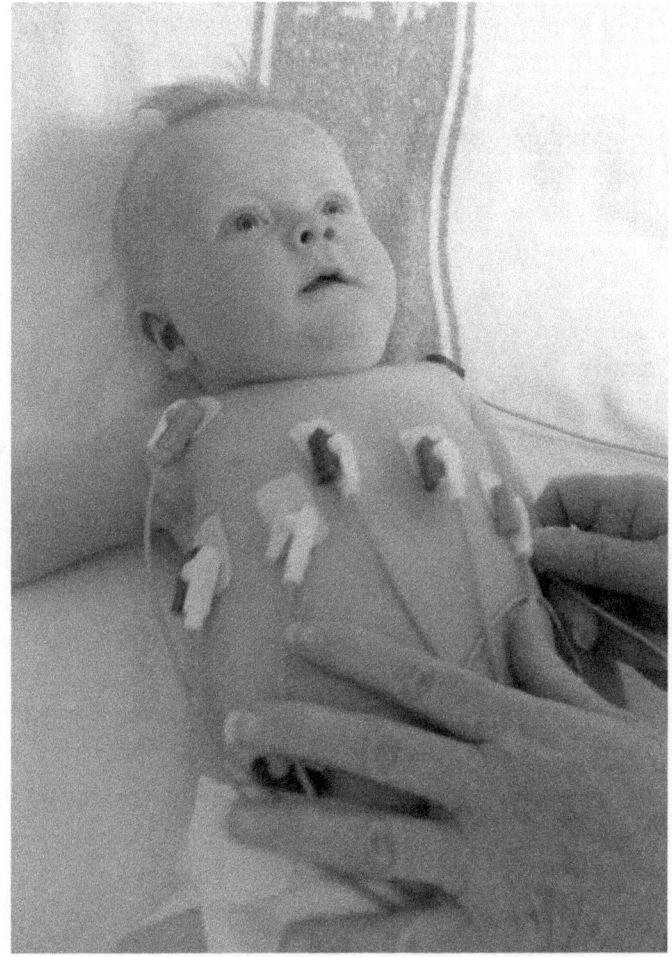

Daniel undergoing an ECG

which test. If you feel comfortable and you wish to know, ask the staff to explain what they are doing. I found that most operators were happy to talk in between periods of strict concentration.

After the physical tests are conducted and whilst still in the pre-admission stage, you will need to have an appointment with the anaesthetist, the surgeon and/or your cardiologist. These appointments may or may not occur on the same day. There will be a lot of information to digest before surgery. Ask if you can audio record the appointment on your mobile phone so that you can re-listen to the conversation later. Alternatively, take a notebook and pen and your list of questions.

The pre-admission nurse will usually take you to visit the NICU or PICU, depending on your baby's age. If you are not familiar with this area, the nurse can show you around and introduce you to the staff. It is important for you to know where to go after surgery and the locations of the ward clerk and parent room, as well as what facilities are available and what you might expect to see when your baby returns from theatre.

Some hospitals use paging systems and mobile devices to notify families when surgery is complete, others will contact you on your mobile phone. Either way, you will be advised during pre-admission how you will be kept informed of your baby's progress while you are separated.

Once the pre-admission list has been ticked off, you will usually have some time to enjoy your baby before having to return to hospital. Admission day can be long and tiring. Try to make sure you have snacks and drinks for you and your baby, not forgetting all the baby items (spare clothes, nappies, the dummy, etc.) and distraction aids to keep him or her as happy as can be throughout the pre-admission process (e.g. toys, rattles and books for baby).

Signing the consent forms is an important and legally necessary part of surgery. This will include information about surgical risks and death. This discussion is confronting but necessary. It may happen during the appointment with your surgeon or it might be done separately in one of those small meeting rooms off the PICU. Either way it is a good idea to consider these issues before the conversation arises. Another important and totally separate topic to raise at some point is organ donation. This is usually only raised if the baby or child is very unwell. This hopefully may never need be a topic that you have to consider, yet it is important for parents to know and understand about the choices concerning organ donation.

The consent form will detail the surgical procedure in medical terminology. This will be explained to you by the surgeon, a fellow or the anaesthetist. Once the form is signed there will likely be a tough conversation about organ donation. You will be asked if you're willing to donate your baby's organs in the event that the surgery is unsuccessful and your baby dies. This is an emotional part of the pre-admission process. Organ donation is a personal choice and there is much literature available via the internet – some may possibly be provided to you in the lead up to this day. Take your time and when you are ready, sign the form. Then practice self-care, which could be going for a walk to reset yourself back into a positive mindset.

Surgery day

Ensure you follow the directions given to you regarding fasting, time of arrival, medications, etc. On average, you are likely to be separated from your baby for about five hours. One thing to consider is that sometimes surgery can and will be cancelled without any prior notice. This can be devastating.

Surgery can be cancelled for many reasons that are out of your control. For example, your baby may become ill in between all the pre-admission testing and this day, your surgeon may be ill, another patient may be prioritised due to an immediate threat to their life, or there may be a shortage of operating theatres, beds or staff in the NICU or PICU. There are so many factors involved for surgery to occur. A cancelled surgery can be devastating after the build-up, especially if you've travelled interstate and left your other children at home. Managing the disappointment and inconvenience of a cancelled surgery may be a bit easier if you are prepared for the possibility.

If surgery is cancelled, you may have to wait to be rescheduled and this may take some time. Try to remember that the doctors would not delay surgery unless it was absolutely necessary. Remember that your baby can live for years while in heart failure.

If surgery is going ahead, the wait for your baby to be taken to theatre can be excruciating. You will often arrive very early in the morning to wait in a large area with other children, all with various medical issues and all nervously awaiting theatre. Make sure you bring toys to distract your baby as well as comfort items. Babies are often required to fast before theatre so make sure you bring aids to distract them from their hunger. As a general rule, the youngest babies are generally sent to theatre first but not always.

A nurse will guide you through the last minute checks such as height, weight, oxygen saturations and blood pressure. Just prior to surgery, the anaesthetist will explain their role to you and sometimes the surgeon may speak to you before the operation commences.

You will then be instructed to put on a protective gown that covers your clothes, shoes and hair. These are to keep the theatre sterile. You will need to follow a staff member to the theatre and physically hand your baby over to a total stranger very soon. Only one adult is permitted to carry the baby to theatre for the handover – this is to minimise germs in theatre. This is a tough part of the day and it won't be the only time you have to go through a handover. Take a deep breath. Be guided by the theatre staff and try to keep yourself calm to protect your baby from picking up your stress. Remember, you are handing your baby over to a team of highly trained professionals who are aiming for a successful surgery. Once you leave the theatre it is okay to cry (well it is really okay at any time you feel the urge). You will be escorted back to the main waiting area and will be free to go from there.

Whilst your baby is in theatre, a new challenge presents itself. Waiting! This can be excruciating and scary. Consider how you might want to spend this time. It may be a good opportunity to eat a meal or have a rest. You may consider other self-care options such as soaking in a hot bath, reading a book, going for a walk, or visiting a chapel. Consider this in advance and plan for what you may need to pack in the hospital bag to help you get through the waiting. A disposable vomit bag is a handy option too if you aren't already carrying one.

At some point, someone from theatre or the intensive care unit will contact you to bring you up to date with progress and when you can see your baby. Follow their instructions.

If you were an inpatient on the morning of surgery (meaning you never got to go home prior to stage one, or you contracted a virus or other complication and were in hospital on this morning), your experience will be slightly different to the description above. Your baby will already be occupying a space in the NICU. This may or may not be the same place your baby will return to after the surgery but you will be notified.

Very early that morning there will be lots of checks being done by the doctors and nurses in the NICU. The anaesthetist will come and talk to you and may insert some of the hardware into your baby's body, prior to transportation to theatre.

You may also notice the nurses preparing drips and bags of fluid, monitoring your baby's blood pressure, and measuring height and weight again. The large trolley bed that transported your baby to the NICU after birth may also be used to transport baby to theatre. All the same tests will be repeated, but this time you will not have to go through the pre-admission clinic or sit in the queue with the other patients awaiting theatre. At some stage a ward person will arrive to push the trolley bed to theatre. You will usually be permitted to accompany your baby to a certain point where you will be afforded a period of time to say goodbye to your baby and exit the area. This experience is never easy. Enjoy the last cuddle.

Post-surgery

Seeing your baby in a post-op state can be confronting and upsetting. Take a breath and move slowly as all the attachments and machinery that you see are keeping your baby stable and allowing recovery to take place. The equipment will become familiar to you over time. If you are interested, ask one of the nurses to explain which apparatus is serving which function. Write it down, sketch a drawing or do what you can to understand what

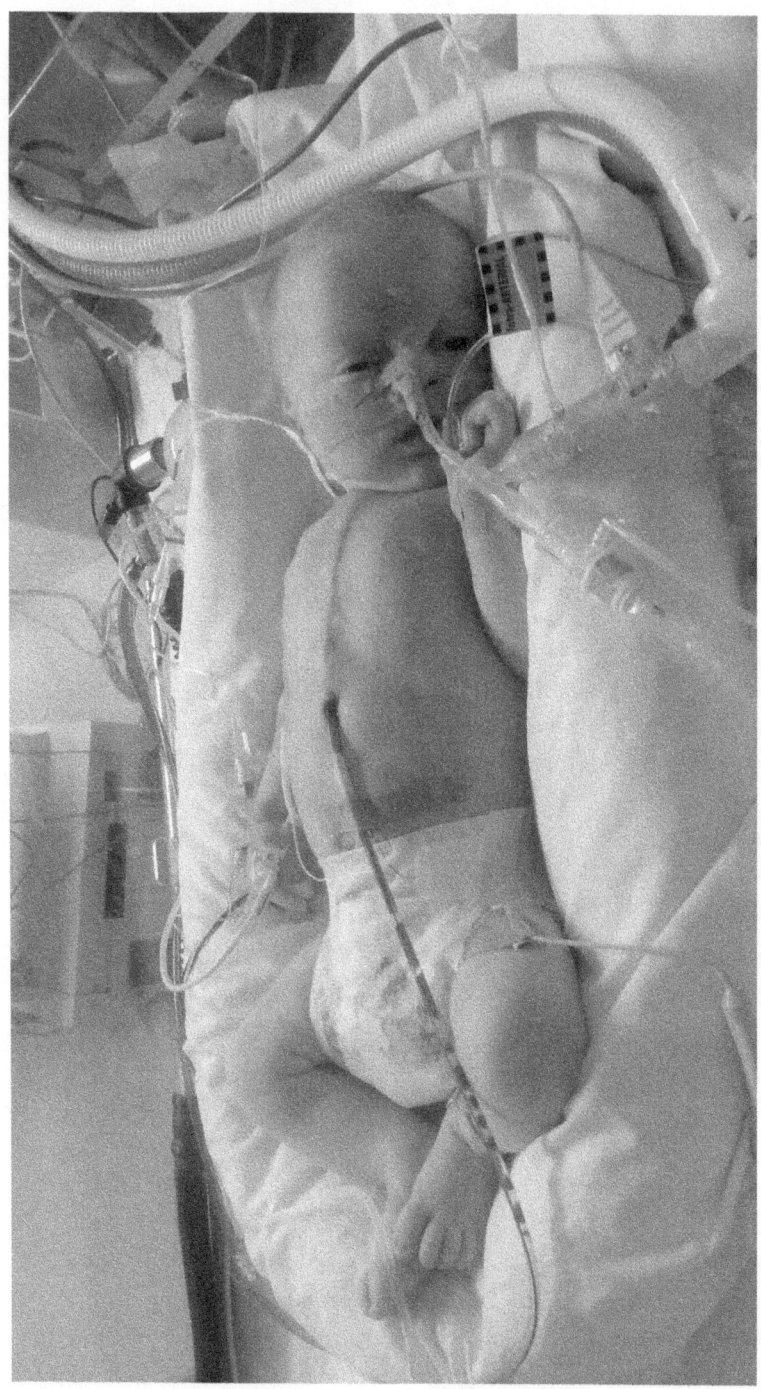

Daniel recovering from his 1st heart surgery the Pulmonary Artery Banding

is going on around you. Try to be aware of your emotions, practice self-care, lean on the support of your team and seek out a social worker if you feel the need. There are people around to support you through this challenging experience.

It is unlikely that you will be allowed to touch or pick up your baby at this stage. Finding any skin that is free from attachments can be a challenge when your baby is so small and it seems like their entire body is connected to something that is beeping. If permitted, find an available patch of skin and gently stroke your baby to soothe them and let them know that you are near. Talk to them – your familiar voice will be comforting. Singing and reading are also good options. Underneath all those attachments, your baby is recovering. He or she will usually only be lying in a nappy without any clothing; this allows the nurses and doctors to access the attachments and tubes, and clear vision for them to conduct their observations and notice any changes.

Each parent will notice different things when they see their baby post-op. I will describe the minimum in this chapter. If things didn't go to plan in theatre, you may see more than what I am about to describe. You are likely to notice the incision on your baby's sternum, the breathing tube, the overhead monitors and various wires. Take a moment to gather yourself together before you get too close to your baby in case you lose your nerve or break down in tears. The good news is that your baby is going to be okay and surgery is complete for now.

The breathing tube may look and sound enormous, it will remain in place until your baby no longer needs it. The tube is attached to the end of baby's nose and connects to a large machine that is breathing for your baby while they recover from surgery. The tube is taped to your baby's face to keep it in place.

The nurses will be extremely busy and actively working to support your baby. It is important to allow them to do their work so keep out of their way. If you're not coping with the sight of your post-op baby practise self-care. Consider taking yourself for a walk while the nurses get everything organised. Neither the nurses nor your baby will benefit from your distress. Your baby will be heavily sedated and will not be affected if you leave the room to calm yourself. Come back when things have settled – a lot can change in a short time. The nurses know what they are doing and will provide the best intensive care available. There is nothing you can do for your baby right now other than stay calm and collected, this situation is out of your control.

You may notice a "central line", sometimes referred to as a jugular line as it is inserted into the jugular vein in the neck. The central line distributes medications and fluid to the rest of the body at speed.

You will see a "pleural drain" poking out of your baby's abdomen which will be connected to an instrument situated somewhere nearby. The pleural drain removes excess blood from the wound in the centre of the chest. Above this drain you will see the surgical incision which will be covered by a sticky layer of protection to prevent infection. This is called a "median sternotomy" and initially it is a horrible-looking red wound. Eventually it will turn into a scar and fade in colour to almost match the skin. Sometimes the doctor will access the heart from the side of the body instead. In some cases, the baby's chest is left open after surgery due to complications such as swelling of the heart. In these cases, the beating heart muscle is visible and heavily protected by special coverings. Your cardiologist or surgeon will usually discuss this possibility with you pre-surgery.

You may notice a "catheter" inserted into the penis/urethra to drain urine. This is useful as it eliminates the need for nappy changes or toileting.

There will be attachments inserted into each of your baby's hands. One of these is likely to be an "arterial line" which looks like a clear plastic tube inserted into the skin at the back of the hand. This line is used to directly monitor blood pressure and to obtain samples for arterial blood gas analysis (another procedure you will become familiar with over time). The other hand will a have a cannula which is inserted through the skin, into a vein, on the top of the hand. The cannula is used to

PULMONARY ARTERY BANDING OR SHUNT

administer fluids and medication and can also be used to obtain blood samples. You will notice that doctors and nurses continually arrive and disappear, taking measurements, making records, and administering medications. Lots of notes are made, sometimes on handwritten charts, but generally via laptop computer.

Depending on your surgeon's schedule, you may get the opportunity to meet with him or her to discuss how things went in theatre and the anticipated plan from this point on. If not the surgeon, someone else from the cardiac team should provide you with information. You may or may not see your surgeon again during this hospital visit (they are extremely busy people and if not them, someone else from their team will be monitoring progress, recovery and reporting back to them).

The longer the breathing tube stays in place, the more often it may need to be suctioned and cleaned out by the nursing team. Your baby may look as if they're trying to cough and this coughing may seem to be due to the tube being in place. Each baby will come out of sedation in their own unique way. Try to keep your baby comfortable and resting while their body recovers from this huge event.

Your baby may cycle through periods of appearing cranky, stable, upset and even in pain. Voice any concerns with the nurse in charge, you are your baby's advocate.

The chest drain is usually removed within 24 hours. The breathing tube will be removed (extubated) as soon as possible. When the breathing tube is removed, it is often replaced with another form of oxygen support (from high flow, to low flow and eventually room air when things are really looking good). You should notice that your baby is more alert by now and spending greater lengths of time awake.

This period can be a worrying time while you sit and observe the nurses going about their business and keeping a close eye out for post-operative infections or other issues. Large teams of doctors and specialists will visit the bedside each day to report and discuss progress. If you have any questions, make sure you use this time to speak to the relevant people.

As each day passes and your child becomes stronger, more of the lines and attachments will be removed. Feeding and a cuddle will hopefully become an option soon. As this will be an emotional experience be prepared with tissues. You may be able to play soft, calming music to your baby. Check with the nurse if this is ok and consider whether it might disturb other babies nearby. You are often in a large room with other babies, their visiting families, and all the staff that continually clock on and off duty. It may be useful to research and think about other possibilities to soothe your baby.

Eventually the staff will advise when you can bathe your baby (this might be the first ever if you haven't yet been home). This can be a comforting and enjoyable experience, both relaxing and exhausting for baby. Enjoy it and don't forget the camera.

Another echo will be conducted post-op. The equipment might be brought to the NICU or you may have to attend the cardiology department within the hospital. One little tip: ask the nurse for sucrose to help keep baby still during the echo. Sucrose is provided in some hospitals in a very small dose which can be placed onto the dummy to soothe and distract baby. It is a sweet option and good source of encouragement for your baby to suck that dummy all the while lying still and complying with the operator.

The echo will be performed by either the cardiologist, a fellow or another trained operator. Ask if it is okay to breastfeed your baby during this test and for any tips on how to get your baby into a good position and how to remain still, which can be challenging if they are hungry or upset.

Most babies will commence taking medications post-op and are likely to still be taking some when it is time to go home. The cardiologist will prescribe a diuretic to keep fluid away from the heart. They will explain administration and doses for your baby as necessary.

PULMONARY ARTERY BANDING OR SHUNT

Hopefully now it's time to go home, rest and recover and enjoy your newborn. Your baby will have further appointments with a paediatrician or cardiologist. You will have been provided guidelines regarding observations of your baby, medications, etc. Make sure you have contact details for your team.

You may also want to consider commencing a daily feeding diary for your baby (depending on your level of exhaustion and or interest). I found this a useful way to track breastfeeds, the length of time a feed took, quantity of daily nappies, hours of sleep and anything else that you may feel is useful as a record. I used this tool to track heart failure and changes in behaviour further along the journey.

LIVING WITH HALF A HEART

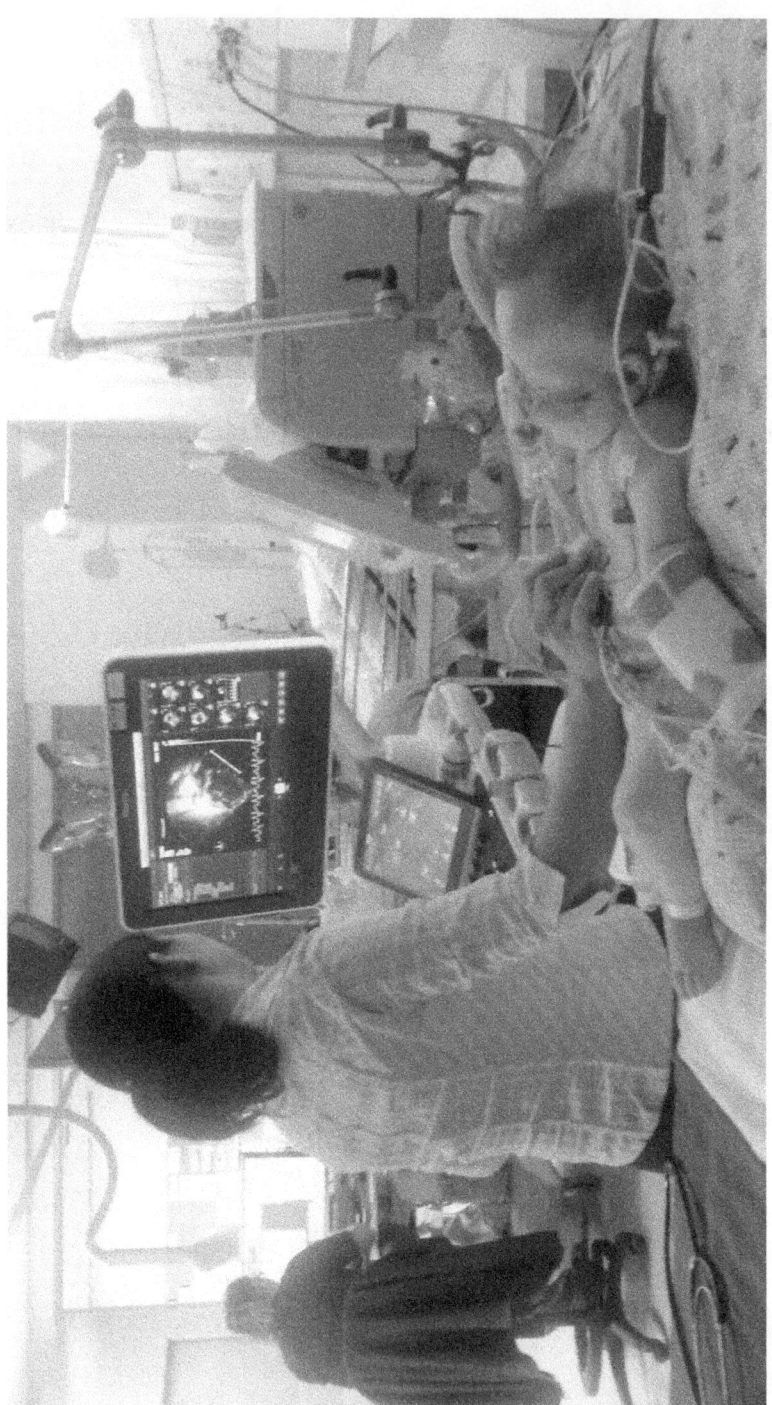

Daniel undergoing an echo on his heart

7.

BIDIRECTIONAL GLENN SHUNT

This second stage of your surgical plan will include open heart surgery on your baby. The purpose of the Bidirectional Glenn Shunt is to get a sufficient amount of blood to the lungs. Your surgeon or cardiologist may or may not describe their plan and actions to you in technical terms (that probably depends on how much of the technical stuff you want to ask for and what your brain at this stage of the game is able to process). Remember your team know what they are doing and everyone has their own role to play in supporting your baby.

In Lib's words, this surgery starts by removing the band that was placed around the pulmonary artery in the first operation. The surgeon will then join your baby's main upper body vein (the superior vena cava) to their right pulmonary artery. This means that the deoxygenated blood travelling back from the head and upper body will go directly to the lungs for oxygenation (instead of going to the heart first to be pumped into the lungs). This will take some of the workload off that single ventricle. The procedure allows the blood to travel "bi-directionally" to both right and left lungs after surgery. The Glenn affords your baby some more time to grow and develop in preparation for Fontan surgery at a later stage.

This is another major medical event and you will need to go through the same pre-admission steps as you did for the banding/shunt in stage one. Some of your baby's medications may need to be stopped prior to surgery but all that information will be discussed with you prior to arriving at this point. You will have been given a plan but be aware that this may change at any time depending on your baby's progress.

This is a major surgery and the risks remain high, but hopefully you will see some familiar faces in the NICU or PICU this time around. You might like to refer back to the list of items that may be handy to pack in your hospital bag for this occasion. While most babies will remain in hospital somewhere between 7–14 days after the Glenn (all going well) each baby's recovery is individual and it may take longer. You may endure a cancellation or your baby may not yet require this surgery (as sometimes they simply take longer to outgrow the first stage of the shunt or band).

If your experience with the hospital has not been great so far, you may wish to try to sort out any problems well in advance of this surgery. Talk to your cardiologist, plan well and do whatever you can to avoid any additional and unnecessary stress.

Prior to arriving at this point, you may have enjoyed a lull in the surgical program. Hopefully life afforded you some precious time for you and your baby to bond and enjoy some living.

Some babies may not have had a chance to go home yet. They may be in and out of hospital or kept in isolation in preparation for surgery. Sadly, some heart-babies will have died before arriving at the Glenn stage.

This period in between the first two surgeries provides you with a short time to prepare better. This time can pass quickly and you may feel like you've barely unpacked your hospital bag before you are searching for it again. While many things are similar in planning for the Glenn, the obvious difference is that your baby is likely to be about six months of age and full of personality. Hopefully he or she will have enjoyed a home and life routine and are eating and sleeping well. Enjoy these periods.

Have a think about how you can best prepare for another surgery and how you might maintain your baby's health and strength. What other players in your team can you engage with to make the next two surgeries go as smoothly as possible and enable maximum recovery? What services or practitioners do you believe in or engage with? What other methods are you prepared to try? You may have also had the chance to network with some other heart mums in your local area or via social media. There's a wealth of knowledge and information shared within these groups if you're interested and have the energy.

During the downtime between surgeries, you may wish to consider seeing a counsellor or psychologist to talk through what's already happened or to help you prepare for the next surgery. Your self-care is high priority going into stage two as there is still a long and stressful road to travel.

You may wish to consider engaging a dietician or naturopath to help boost your baby's immune system. Some families report benefits from supplements such as zinc, vitamin A & D, or cod liver oil, others endorse probiotics.

Personally, my recommendation, based on my own experience, is osteopathy. Osteopathy is a non-invasive treatment and something that I believe has had a big impact on my baby's health, his recovery from all surgeries and his general wellness and overall function. Some osteopaths focus on working with newborns. I felt that our osteopath was able to improve body function in my son, especially supporting his precious young heart and respiratory system. There was obvious relief witnessed as well as better sleep patterns following successive treatments.

I cannot say that this second surgery is easier than the first – it is not. Your baby is now older and carrying him or her down to the operating theatre is a new experience because your child is not that newborn that snuggled into your neck as you walked the corridor previously. Your child will be older, more aware and with more capacity to pick up on your own stress and anxiety. Expect to be confronted by that ugly consent form again. Just like your first pre-admission experience, you will have appointments with your team members prior to theatre. Make sure your questions are answered and you feel prepared.

Baths for your baby will be off limits after surgery until the drains have been removed. So if you and your baby enjoy bath time together, make sure you schedule this in before heading back to hospital. Self-care is also important, please consider how you can best prepare yourself for the next surgery. You might consider a massage, hydrotherapy float, or a visit to a day spa. Remember, hospital stays are stressful and exhausting so enjoy your time at home while you can.

The pre-admission clinic will include all the standard pre-theatre tests, measurements of height, weight, blood pressure, oxygen saturations, temperature, and ECG, echo and so on. Follow the guidelines provided and get that checklist ticked off.

Another point worth raising and checking with your cardiologist is your baby's immunisations, especially if these fall around the time of the planned surgery for the Glenn. Sometimes the immunisations are deferred due to the need for your baby to be on bypass during theatre and/or undergoing a blood transfusion. It is worth the conversation and adding to your list of questions.

Once the pre-admission requirements have been satisfied and your theatre date is finalised you will have a short period to enjoy your baby before you need to report to the designated area in preparation for theatre.

As before, basic checks are conducted and the anaesthetist will come and speak with you to go through the process. To reduce stress for an older baby, staff may ask you to administer the medication to make your baby drowsy. If so, this is administered orally. It is standard procedure that only one parent escorts the baby to theatre. Be prepared for the mask to

BIDIRECTIONAL GLENN SHUNT

be placed over your baby's face, this is the gas that puts them to sleep. You may be permitted to nurse your baby throughout this process. It's challenging to give them that last hug and say goodbye. It is a further challenge to walk away from the theatre. You'll be escorted back to the main waiting area while the surgery is performed and the Glenn shunt is put into place. Try to look after yourself during this wait. It's a tough time but can be a good chance for a rest, a walk, a decent meal or whatever gets you through.

The same system as in stage one surgery is likely to follow. Someone from the NICU, PICU or theatre team will contact you to advise when you can see your baby and where to go. At some stage soon after surgery, someone from the team, hopefully the surgeon, will meet with you to advise what happened in theatre and if surgery went according to plan.

It's confronting to see your child on the bed in the PICU after this surgery. I found it to be a different experience from the stage one surgery (probably because he had grown so much in between surgeries and my child seemed so big in his body). I was very aware that he was back in the recovery phase and I felt the unfairness for him to have to relive this pain again. It was hard to see or even find one patch of skin that didn't feel like it was covered with a tube, monitoring patch, drain, etc. It's confronting and I wasn't really prepared to see this again nor did I want him to have to go through this all again. I am unsure if you can prepare for some of the feelings and emotions that may arise in you. Go gently.

When you arrive at intensive care, be prepared to see your baby surrounded by people. They'll be attending to all the required duties in this early post-operative period. Don't be confronted by the number of them, they'll come and go and eventually reduce in number.

You may notice the breathing tube attached to baby's nose and the large, noisy machine. The tube runs from your baby's trachea out to the ventilator, which is a large machine allowing your baby to rest and take a break from having to breathe on his/her own. This may or may not be familiar to you from the first surgery.

After the stage one surgery, you will recall having seen one chest drain coming out from your baby's tummy. The Glenn procedure sees three chest drains coming out from the midsection. All of these have blood and fluids that drain into containers, which are stored on the floor close to the bedside. Those three containers are monitored and recorded often by the nursing team.

Two of the drains are "mediastinal", meaning that they're in the middle of the chest. The third drain is a "pleural drain", meaning it sits in the space around the lungs. The three drains will be taped down to your baby's tummy. They're ugly but not painful. The contents of the drains are visible so try not to look if you're not good with blood and fluid. Draining is a good thing and the nurse will keep a very close eye on the drains and their output.

Another item you will notice is a "cannula", it might be in the foot or elsewhere depending on the set-up. The cannula is really handy and is an item used for many purposes, but initially to give extra fluid. The foot or wrist will house the little ID bracelet that has your baby's name, date of birth, treating doctor and hospital number. This will be checked often, especially before administering any medications.

There is likely to be a variety of equipment attached to the body. The left arm may house the familiar "arterlia line" which is taped down to a small pad inside the forearm. Staff use this line to measure the pressure in the veins and give a continuous reading of blood pressure.

Somewhere on the body (often a finger or toe) is the "oxygen saturation probe". This provides a continuous reading of the level of oxygen in your baby's blood. The probe can be a source of irritation for some babies. My son was an expert at removing this item from whichever location the nurses tried. It is usually taped to a finger or toe and can be easily dislodged with movement. Every baby will have their own "normal" with regard to oxygen levels prior to Fontan surgery. It is not unusual for babies with CHD to saturate in the 70s or even lower. If you have any concerns about the numbers, please ask your cardiologist or the nurse on duty.

BIDIRECTIONAL GLENN SHUNT

One of the other things that you'll become familiar with post-surgery and during any hospital admission are the small red/black plastic dot monitoring devices that are stuck to the chest of your child. These monitor different readings within the chest such as heart rate and pulse.

The "central line" will be on the right hand side of your baby's neck. This transports medications straight into the jugular vein and it is a very handy apparatus.

You may notice another wire on one of your baby's legs: this is the "rectal thermometer" that is inserted into the anus. This provides staff with a constant temperature and will be removed when appropriate.

Like in the previous surgery, you may also notice another cannula to drain urine. This will be removed when your baby is able to urinate unassisted and without the risk of infection.

You will also see the "nasal gastric" (NG) tube inserted into the nostril. This provides nutrition while feeding is not an option. The quantity of fluids and milk provided are strictly administered and increased throughout this phase of post-operative recovery. The doctor will advise when breast/bottle feeding can resume.

The first few hours post-operation are very busy. It is likely that your baby will need an X-ray and an echo. Doctors and nurses will continually be checking that all wires and tubes are in the right place.

Similar to recovery from the first surgery, there is a fine art to removing the lines, tubes, wires, oxygen, NG tube and so on. It's a process and these trained individuals know exactly what they are doing and are proficient in undertaking the various tasks involved. Try to get some rest and tag team with your support partner. Be guided by the doctors and nurses and always speak up for your baby if you feel there is an issue. You know your baby best.

As your baby recovers, your cardiologist or a nurse educator will advise you about the medications that are required to be taken after going home.

You will also be told how to manage your baby in this period. Because baby is older and possibly even rolling or trying to crawl, this can pose new risks for the sternotomy. There may be a time period discussed where your baby is to refrain from too much movement throughout the chest. This is to protect the stitches and wound and to prevent any complications.

One suggestion is to purchase, borrow or hire some items to keep baby strapped into position, such as a baby rocker, gentle swing or activity mat. The last thing anyone needs is to return to hospital for a reason or incident which could have been avoided. Between feeding and sleeping, I moved my baby from one item to another about every 20–30 minutes while he was awake and when he wasn't in the pram or high chair. It can become challenging after a while but have a think about safe ways in which you can keep baby happy and entertained whilst recovering and protecting the sternotomy. Long walks are a great option for both mum and baby.

Depending on your cardiologist and sometimes even the hospital, your baby will be prescribed blood thinning medications (usually Asprin or Warfarin). Given your baby is now sporting a new shunt, the blood needs to be kept thin and able to move freely around this hardware. Always follow the prescribed medications and discuss any queries with your doctor.

Most babies will go home with a cocktail of medications including diuretics. Keeping an eye on the oxygen saturations is standard practice but by now you will be more relaxed about the changing shades of your baby's cyanosis. It is likely that your baby will still be blue or purple until the next surgery is complete.

For now, it is time to rest and recover once again. Congratulations on making it to the end of stage two.

BIDIRECTIONAL GLENN SHUNT

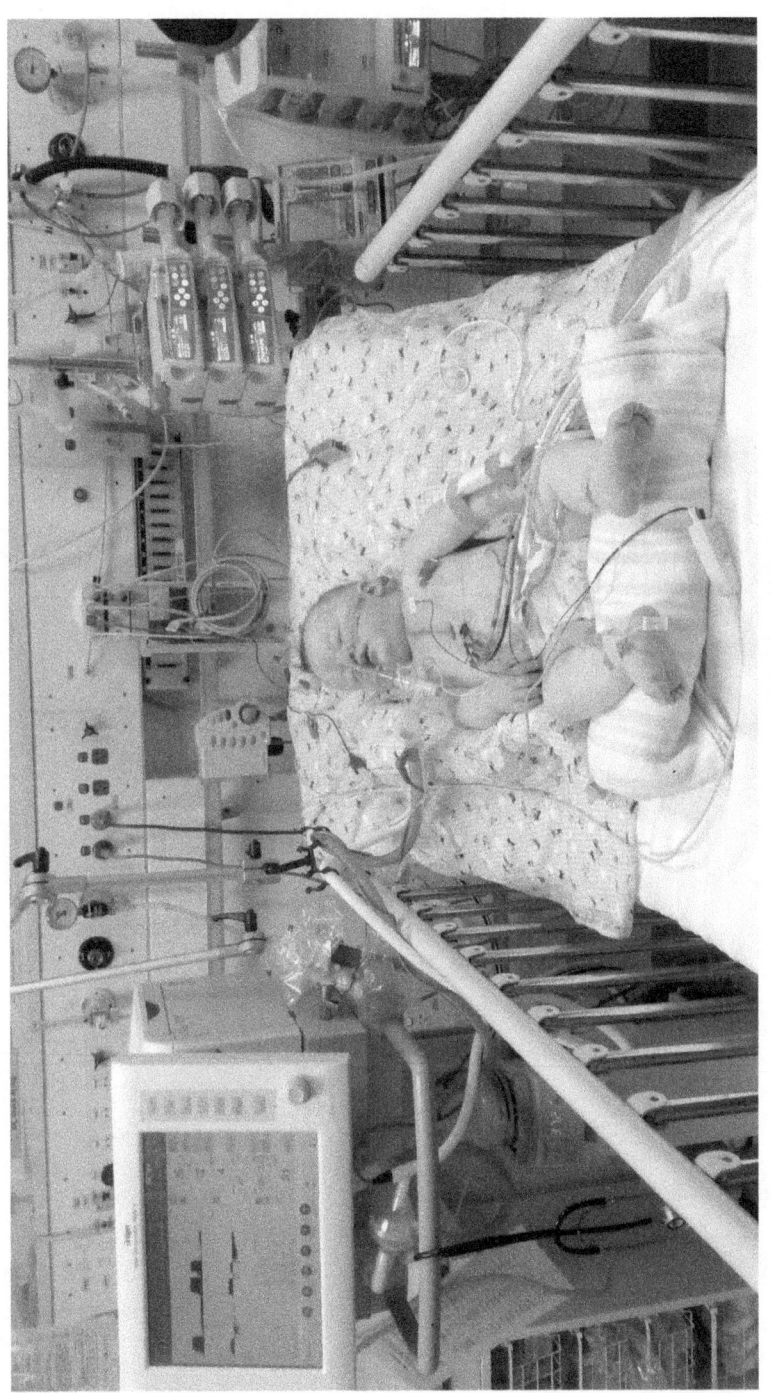

Daniel in the NICU recovering from his Glenn

8.

PREPARATION FOR FONTAN AND FONTAN SURGERY

Prior to the pre-admission phase of preparing for Fontan surgery, it is likely that you will first have to prepare your child and yourself for a visit to the cardiac catheterisation laboratory, also called the "Cath Lab".

Babies will be admitted to hospital either the day before or the morning of the procedure, and they will be required to fast before the procedure. Upon arrival they will be examined by a doctor, an anaesthetist and/or a nurse. Sometimes a blood test will be required. A "mini" version of pre-admission will be conducted and an ECG and X-ray may also be required.

The purpose of this visit to the Cath Lab is to gather information, check pressures within the heart and take pictures. Your child will require another anaesthetic during this appointment, which is usually a day visit or short stay. The Cath Lab information provides vital data for planning the Fontan Surgery. Talk it over with your cardiologist and ask all the questions you have on your mind about the road ahead.

The actual catheter used during the visit to the lab is a fine and flexible tube which is inserted into either a vein or an artery in the groin, arm or neck of your baby. The catheter is guided by the doctor through the heart, main veins and arteries, checking pressures and taking measurements.

A special fluid is injected via the catheter to enable the doctors to see the details of the heart clearly. This is called an "angiogram".

You will not be able to stay with your baby during the Cath Lab visit (similar to a trip to theatre for surgery). Once the procedure is completed, you will be notified either via pager or phone and directed to recovery where you will likely find your baby in a sleepy or groggy state. While some babies undergo the procedure with no adverse effects, others may be affected by the anaesthetic. Having your familiar face, voice and touch for your child upon their waking up from this procedure can greatly assist and provide comfort for them. It can assist the nursing staff too.

One thing to note during this early period of recovery is that you may find yourself in a large space occupied by lots of beds and varying ages of children from all types of procedures. The area can fill up and be emptied depending on the length of time you spend in recovery and how long before your own bed is prepared on the ward or elsewhere. The reaction of other children and noise level in this space can be confronting. Not all children are supported by a parent or family member. Be prepared to focus on the needs of your little one to assist him or her to recover as soon as possible. It is noisy, busy and can be challenging.

Another note to point out is that by the time your Cath Lab visit arrives, your baby will be older than previous visits to hospital. He or she may now be a toddler and may be placed on a ward instead of the PICU. You will find that the ward operates in a very different manner under a different set-up, daily operation and conditions. The ward can be busier and noisier than the PICU with children of older and wider ranges of ages. It can be a good experience to spend some time on the ward at this point on the journey, especially if this is where you may find yourself transferred to after the actual Fontan Surgery.

You should receive verbal results of the findings following the Cath Lab, usually on the same day. The doctor or fellow will discuss these with you if possible and a written report will follow at a later date. These results will help your surgeon and his team to plan and schedule the Fontan Surgery. You may also be provided with a date for surgery on this day.

Discharge from the Cath Lab will depend on how your child is recovering. Some babies will go home that same day, others may be kept in for one or two nights. Fingers need to be crossed to avoid contracting a virus or bug whilst in the hospital during this visit. Infections or other complications are a distinct possibility so be prepared for this eventuality. Keeping well can be a real challenge while immune systems remain compromised and low.

If the doctor utilised the groin vein during the Cath Lab, you are sure to notice bruising and a small wound in this area. The steristrips covering the wound will need to be removed at home via the instructions provided to you upon discharge. Talk to your doctor about any restrictions following this visit and how to look after the wound. A bruise may or may not develop and spread over the next few days and the area will be tender and even sore. The information gained about your baby's heart during this process is invaluable.

Preparation for Fontan Surgery

For most, the preparation for this open heart surgery has been years in the making. No doubt you will have experienced much and gained a wealth of knowledge, experience and wisdom along the way. You will have also met some of the most talented and gifted humans working within the hospital system and local cardiac world.

As a result, preparing for the Fontan might be seen as "easier" because by now you might consider yourself a "pro" and familiar with the NICU, PICU and the way the hospital, theatre and this entire process operates. You may have even stayed on the ward where all the cardiac patients recover. Whether comfortable or not, preparing to return to hospital can be confronting. This surgery may come with complications and an admission longer than those previously experienced is a possibility.

The pre-admission clinic for Fontan Surgery will include a visit to the nurse, an echo, blood pressure check, a chest X-ray, an ECG and various swabs. These tests might be done the day before the theatre visit or the morning of the visit. Either way you'll have had time to prepare your child. Discuss with your team how much information your child should receive about this surgery. Every hospital will have their own advice and information packs. You know your child best and know how to best communicate with them. Anything you can do to reduce some of the stressors upon waking up after Fontan Surgery is advised. Your child is older now, and he or she will be more capable, more intelligent and more aware of what is about to happen. After surgery he or she will be uncomfortable, confronted with stomach drains and all types of attachments and may even store a conscious memory of this visit and some of the associated pain and challenges.

Some ideas about preparing in advance for this surgery

You may consider a "mock up" or "pretend" Fontan Surgery involving your child as the cardiologist. Draw the zipper on the chest of an old soft toy and open the conversation around why our children have a zipper (the sternotomy scar) and what it is used for. You might place a nappy on the toy if your child is still using nappies and see what other attachments you can make and stitch onto the body of this toy (oxygen mask to put your child to sleep right before theatre, etc.). This can be a fun way to prepare yourself and your child.

The chest drains form a big part of recovery from Fontan Surgery. Most children will wake to discover four separate chest drains poking out of

PREPARATION FOR FONTAN AND FONTAN SURGERY

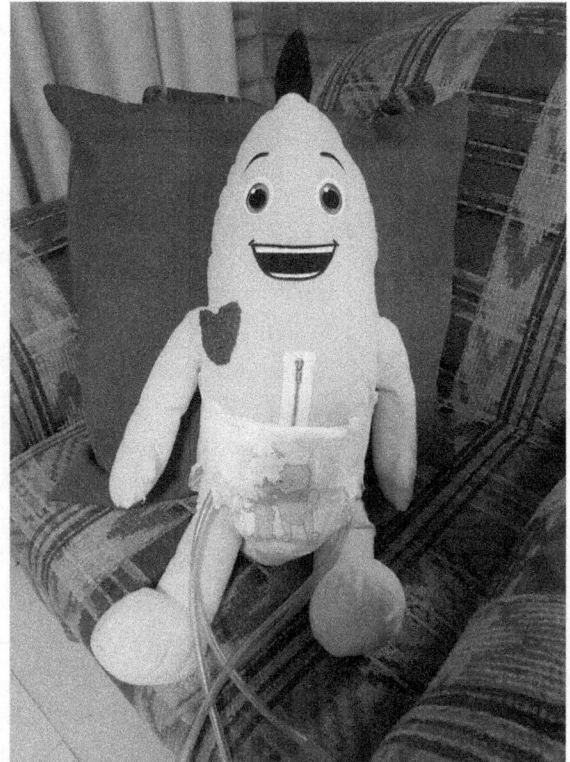

The banana who lost his pyjamas and inherted a dextrocardia, a zipper, nappy and chest drains

their abdomen. Although these are not painful, they are uncomfortable and make sleep and movement in the early post operation days somewhat problematic. Ask if your child can physically touch and feel a similar drain before they undergo surgery, as this can help reduce the impact of the sight of the drains post-surgery. The doctors and nurses pay very strict attention to these drains and the recording of their output with regular tapping of the drains (so they don't clog up). Whatever you can do to help your child to be comfortable with their presence, feel or sight will be very beneficial.

Another fun idea when preparing for this visit and potentially a longer hospital stay is the creation of an "incentive box" for your child (maybe hidden from the child initially until you need to make use of it post-surgery). Shopping for small items to gift to your child can be one way of helping to provide a distraction or a reward for participation in the blood tests, physiotherapy, drain removal, etc. When an incentive to participate is needed, this box can be a godsend.

Some good resources written by parents of Fontan recipients, and also hospital resources, exist and can be highly beneficial for your child and yourself. Start reading hospital stories with your child and their siblings in preparation for this event. You will know the timing best but a wide range of resources are available in standard public libraries.

The day of your Fontan Surgery

Only one parent will be able to take the child to theatre. Your child might be given a liquid sedation (also referred to as a "pre-med"). This will assist in getting your little one off to sleep quickly. A gown, hat and shoe coverings are needed to cover your clothing and keep germs to a minimum before you start your walk with an escort to the operating theatre. You will have experienced this feeling before but this time may be different as your child is older and perhaps more aware. Your child might be permitted to walk into the area and receive the sedation medication in the prep room. Alternatively, you may be asked to nurse the child while the mask and gas are placed over their face to send them off to sleep. At some stage your child will be sedated and they will feel limp and heavy. You will be asked to lie the child onto the bed, say a quick goodbye and then leave the room.

The walk back to the outside world and the nervous wait begins until the pager, beeper or your mobile phone rings to advise you that surgery is over. There will be hours of waiting and the wait can be horrendous. Remember your self-care as your baby will be receiving plenty of attention.

9.

RECOVERING FROM FONTAN SURGERY

THE RECOVERY PERIOD VARIES for each child. You may be provided an anticipated timeframe to remain in hospital post-op, however this can change without notice. Hospital stays can vary from two weeks to two months or longer, often depending on when the chest drains cease draining. Your team or cardiologist will advise you as best they can.

When your child is well enough, they will be transferred to an area for recovery. This might be the NICU, PICU or the ward. Your child will have lots of attachments and you will be familiar with most of these from the previous surgeries. The chest drains, pressure lines, pacing wires and breathing tube will confront you once again. When you arrive in the recovery area, hopefully you will see your child comfortable, relaxed and sleeping. Parents are not usually allowed in to visit until the child is set up in recovery and ready for your arrival.

Your child is likely to be really thirsty when they wake up, but fluid intake is restricted during early recovery to reduce the risk of fluid collecting in the lungs or elsewhere. This thirst can be tough on children and their request for a drink can be continuous and challenging. Special sponges that look like a lollipop (and are lodged on the end of a plastic stick) are offered to moisten your child's lips and can provide lubrication. The fluid restriction will be decreased over time as your child recovers.

Various tests will be conducted in the short term, such as an echo, ECG and X-ray. You may only notice your baby open their eyes briefly before exhaustion sets in and they fall back to sleep again. Sometimes the breathing tube can impact the vocal cords and make speaking difficult, and the voice may change temporarily too. You probably experienced all this before when your child underwent the Bidirectional Glenn Shunt at stage two.

Many observations and records are maintained by the staff, including keeping a close eye on the output from the chest drains. Similar to the previous surgery, the attachments will be removed when the time is right. Don't hesitate to speak to the teams, nurses or administration staff with any queries.

Physiotherapy is an important and ongoing part of recovery. Lots of bubble blowing and popping will help to open the lungs and encourage movement. Initially, your baby may not want to see the physiotherapist or participate in the activities but their resistance will ease over time as they start to feel stronger and experience less pain. Physiotherapy can be exhausting and excruciating and sometimes it feels like it never ends. Your support plays an important role in your child's participation and recovery. Try to be positive and supportive of the staff, it will benefit your child's recovery and remember they feed off you.

Four chest tubes will assist with clearing blood from the heart and abdomen. These are called the mediastinal drain, right pleural drain, left pleural drain and the peritoneal (abdominal) drain. All four tubes and their contents are visible. You can see them draining fluid from your

RECOVERING FROM FONTAN SURGERY

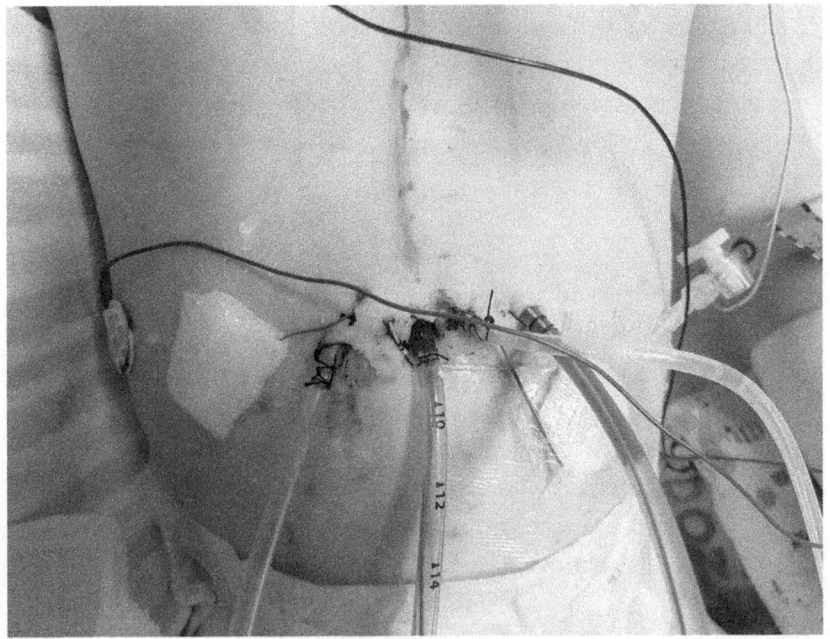

Daniel's four chest drains and zipper

child's body at different rates. When the nurses are not too busy, they're usually happy to tell you about the attachments and their role in recovery from Fontan surgery.

Some of the other visible attachments include the arterial line, central line, catheter, oxygen saturation monitor and pacing wires. Clearing out the breathing tube is an unpleasant and regular event for your child around this time. The nurses will clear the tube when necessary to keep the lines clear of secretions and working well. Sometimes the physiotherapists will assist with this. A blocked tube can be uncomfortable for your child. The physiotherapist will encourage regular coughing to promote recovery. You will note that every hour and day post-operation should get easier for your child, so just hang in there.

If all is going well, about 24–48 hours post-surgery, it is likely that your child will be transferred from the PICU to the ward. This transfer signals the start of the recovery process but the timing will also depend on bed availability.

The fluid restrictions should decrease as your child starts to eat and drink more. All these signs are positive. The draining will continue and can happen quickly or slowly. One or two drains may have been removed in the first week post-op. Drains are removed one at a time and not usually on the same day.

Once some of the attachments have been removed, the physiotherapist will be keen to get your child out of bed and moving around, with or without drains and attachments. This may seem like an impossible task and a major increase in expectation from blowing bubbles in bed. But movement aids recovery. You should feel comfortable to ask questions and raise concerns with the physiotherapist. It's tough to see your child in pain as they try to take a few exhausting steps, but these exercises are a critical part of recovery and your help is important. The easier and more fun you make this activity, the better and quicker your child's recovery is likely to be.

Medication during this period is likely to include pain relief, sedation, diuretics and potentially an anticoagulant (Warfarin or Aspirin) to prevent blood clots. Sluggish blood flow in the main veins and lung circulation increase the risk of blood clots in these areas or in the heart. While on this drug it is important to remember that your child may bruise easily or bleed for longer than normal after an injury. Your child will likely continue with these medications long-term and may switch between Warfarin and Aspirin at a later stage depending on your cardiologist's advice.

Warfarin has an unpleasant taste and it can be tricky to get kids to swallow the tablet. Ask the nursing staff for tips or try crushing the tablet and hiding it in yoghurt or ice cream. It is a good idea to practice administering medication while still in hospital given that you will be responsible for medication administration after discharge. If your child refuses the tablet or spits it out, ask the nurse for the liquid option.

Your child may require another ECG, echo or Magnetic Resonance Imaging (MRI) if draining is slow and delays their recovery. The equipment will be brought to the bedside when possible, otherwise transport to other areas in the hospital will be coordinated and you will be escorted by a nurse for the majority of the time.

You may see your child behaving differently – they may be angry, unfriendly and non-compliant. Remember that staff don't take this personally and most will get the task done as quickly as possible to reduce further distress. This is all perfectly normal, so roll with the recovery and all the ups and downs and just do your best to support your little one.

It is likely that your child will be moved to different beds or even different rooms on the ward. Initially, your child might be placed close to the nurse's station and gradually moved further away as their immediate care needs decrease. You may be moved onto a ward with additional roommates. The extra noise and people can be challenging but this change provides an opportunity to make new friends and increase the fun times.

You may be seen by a dietician depending on how your child's drainage is progressing and whether there are any issues that can be boosted by supplements or a special diet. If required or necessary, this will be communicated to you. Your child will be weighed daily to help monitor fluid assessment. This can be uncomfortable in the early days when movement is painful and challenging but movement gets easier as pain decreases.

Doctors and nurses will continue to monitor for complications such as pleural effusions (fluid around the lungs), or pericardial effusion (fluid collection around the heart). These may have been discussed with you prior to surgery and if detected will be treated accordingly. Don't hold back to voice any concerns or changes that you notice. You know your child best.

Parents are not usually encouraged to stay overnight in the NICU and PICU and beds for parents are not provided. Most hospitals will provide a chair bedside and some will allow you to stay 24/7 but this needs to be discussed with your team. Once a child is transferred to the ward, a family member is expected to stay overnight and a pull-out bed will be provided. Sleep can be difficult given the routine nursing checks, noisy neighbours, hospital equipment, cleaners, other staff, visitors, volunteers etc. Think about items you can bring to hospital to help you sleep: ear plugs, eye mask, your phone, a headset/earphones, music, guided meditation, audiobooks or a podcast.

Most children will be able to return to normal activity after the first three months post-surgery. There will be doctors checks and communications with your team in the early days of getting home. Most children will be free of cyanosis after this surgery and will have oxygen levels close to normal or hopefully saturating in the 90s.

RECOVERING FROM FONTAN SURGERY

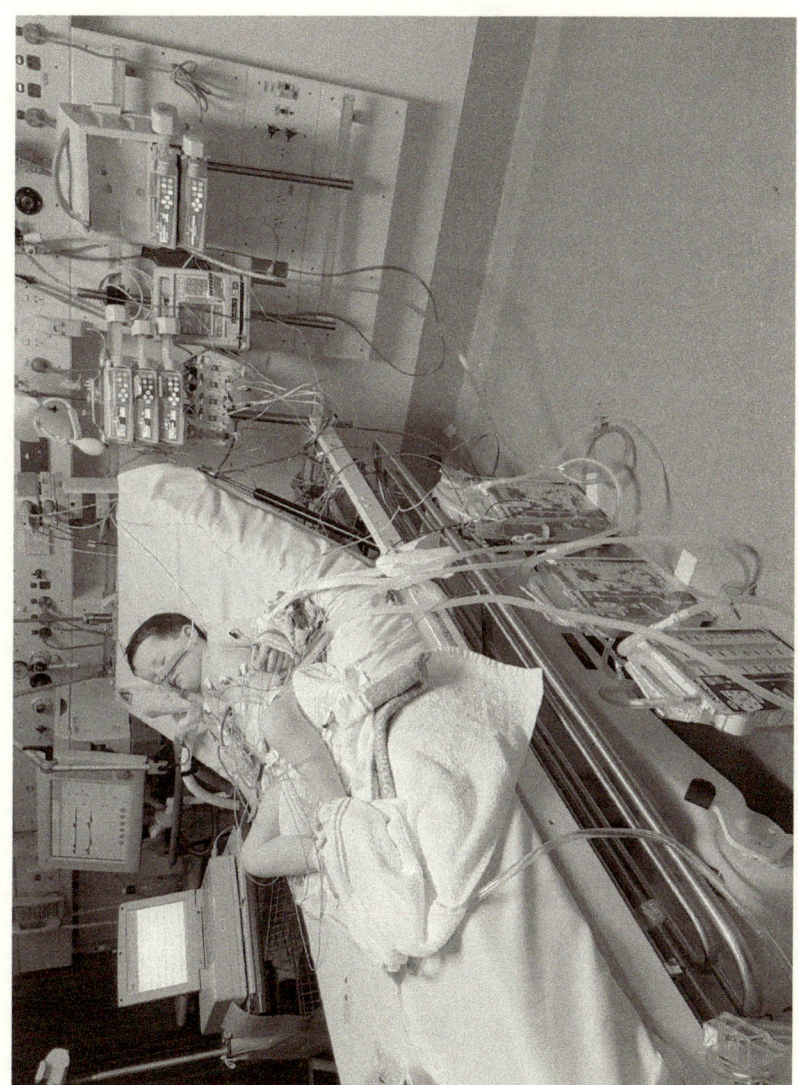

Daniel recovering from his Fontan surgery, see drain storage units on the floor

10.

WRAPPING UP AND GETTING READY

After you finish reading this book, it will soon be time to think about forming your team of trusted people to aid you on the journey ahead. There is stress and challenges before you and your family but this three-staged theatre option is all totally worth it. Don't be afraid to ask for help.

Your baby will need a GP. If possible, seek out someone who has an interest in CHD and experience in this field. Ask your own GP if they have a recommendation. Your baby will need to be examined by a GP upon returning home after surgery, as well as for normal baby reasons. Many GPs will have limited knowledge of and experience with a Fontan circulation.

Your baby's care may be overseen by a paediatrician between cardiology appointments. Your hospital will have a list of practitioners who are experienced in dealing with CHD in newborn babies. Talk to your GP about their recommendations and have someone's details and contact information on hand in case you need it. Paediatricians will generally oversee your baby's progress and work with your GP and cardiologist and other professionals as needed. They can provide relief to you when professionals with knowledge of Fontan surgery are few and far between.

You may be assigned a midwife from the high-risk pregnancy team. Midwives have a wealth of knowledge and practical experience. You can also seek out a midwife at the local level to keep an eye on your progress post-birth.

A paediatric cardiologist works specifically with children with heart conditions. Some work privately and others work in public hospitals. Ask your midwife or GP how you identify which cardiologists are options for you to consider. If, at any time, one of your team doesn't feel right, you have the right to switch them for someone else. It's completely okay to interview a cardiologist prior to engaging their services. It's important to know their experience in dealing with the type of heart defect you are anticipating. Compile a list of questions to ask this person and add to it as the appointment gets nearer.

Your cardiologist will usually line you up with a surgeon, but again you should have a say in who this person is going to be. Research the surgeon's background, ask questions, and make sure they feel like the right fit for your team and your family. These people are extremely important and will be working hard to save your child's life. You need to feel safe in their care and comfortable enough to communicate with them at every level. It is okay to say no, this is your child's life and immediate future.

Consider the topics of retirement, resignation, illness and uncontrollable events that can happen to the people within your team. Professional people can come and go unexpectedly from your team, hopefully with some warning but not always. Be prepared for change when an individual team player may need to leave the equation, especially when you are not expecting or wanting this to occur. If, for example, your surgeon resigns unexpectedly, try not to panic. This doesn't necessarily mean that your child's next surgery won't be successful. Sometimes change is a good thing and replacing one professional for another doesn't mean Fontan circulation won't be achieved. Many things are out of your control in life, so try to adapt to the challenges as best you can.

You will meet many people along this journey, and some of them will be amazing and will assist you in ways that you could not have anticipated. There are lactation consultants, nurses, chaplains, social workers, ward clerks, volunteers and many others. One very important organisation you may become familiar with on this journey is the Ronald McDonald House Charity which supports the families of sick children.

There are 18 Ronald McDonald Houses in Australia, all located in close proximity to the major womens' and childrens' hospitals. The houses provide a homely and inviting place to stay for parents, guardians, carers and siblings of the baby, child or teen undergoing treatment. There are some costs and criteria for eligibility.

At some stage a social worker or nurse may raise this accommodation option with you. They may also give you forms to complete in order to start the booking process. There are small fees for accommodation and a subsidy scheme if you are eligible. Accommodation is always subject to availability and priority is given to families with a recent diagnosis, a seriously injured or sick child, those requiring emergency treatment, families travelling long distances, and mothers experiencing a high-risk pregnancy.

Keeping the family together can be tough when a child is sick and hospital stays are long. Some families stay at a Ronald McDonald House when siblings are brought to the hospital for visits. Each house has a range of accommodation and most include private and common areas. Visitors can receive support and information from in-house staff, volunteers or other families who are sharing similar experiences.

Having a sick child and enduring long hospital stays can be exhausting. It can feel like the outside world no longer exists. These special houses can provide respite for you and a chance for you to take a break and sleep in a real bed, have a hot shower, eat a home-cooked meal, hang out a load of washing or take a walk within the house grounds.

Some of the houses provide external entertainment options and complimentary tickets to local events, tourist attractions and sporting games (usually kindly donated from partners of the charity or the children's hospital). These houses provide the opportunity to reconnect with family and spend precious time together. Having breaks from the bedside, if possible, is important for your mental health and wellbeing. Try to grab a break where possible and look after yourself.

Each of these houses is usually conveniently located and within walking distance to the hospital. A secure place for your vehicle is usually made available (relieving the stress of hospital parking and cost) as is a place to leave your belongings.

The Ronald McDonald Charity in Australia is always busy and active in raising funds. There are annual fundraising days (like McHappy Day at the McDonalds restaurant) and annual walks in major cities trying to raise the profile of the charity and find more supporters and funding. Various programs exist within the hospital systems (like education programs for children on the ward and their siblings) and various respite and holiday homes across this country are also available. Information is readily available via the Ronald McDonald Charity website or through the office at the house in which you are staying. Put this option on your list to check out prior to the birth of your baby as pregnant mothers prior to induction are also welcome to stay as guests.

WRAPPING UP AND GETTING READY

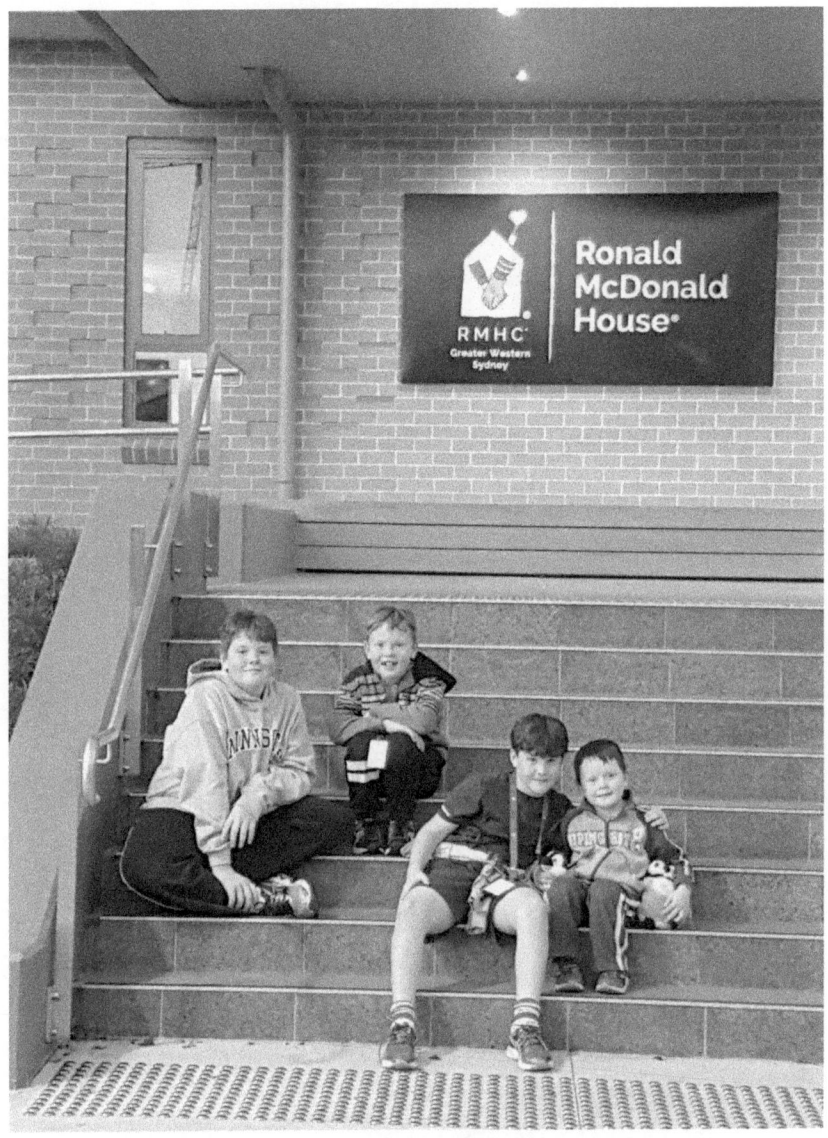

**The house that love built, thank you Ronald McDonald Charity.
L-R John, Stuart, Matthew, Daniel and his penguin**

CONCLUSION AND A LIFELONG COMMITMENT TO YOUR BABY AND THEIR CHD

My aim throughout these chapters was to cover the anticipated journey for you and your baby with a CHD. This started with your diagnosis right through to leaving hospital after Fontan surgery. At minimum, this included:

- Your antenatal experience and the remaining 20 weeks of your pregnancy
- The birth of your precious baby
- Pre-surgery and the wait for Stage One (banding/shunt)
- Stage Two being the Bidirectional Glenn Shunt and the waiting game in between surgery
- Fontan completion and recovery (Stage Three).

Getting through these phases and early years of your baby's life is a massive accomplishment for both you and your child and the whole family. Of course the journey will not end there as once life settles down and your child develops and hopefully thrives with their new circulation, there will be further hurdles with challenges and even more joyous reasons to appreciate every single day.

By the time your baby has developed into a five or six-year-old, you'll be confronted with the idea of starting school and how that will change your life as you have experienced it. Each child will be tracking in their own unique style and schooling will bring about an increase in physical, mental and social challenges and delights too.

Further to this and about seven years after commencing formal schooling, there will be the issues surrounding navigating the teenage years. Having a Fontan circulation can be limiting and isolating (for some but not all). Teenagers having been through the trauma of early surgeries may be affected in various ways which can present additional challenges in this 21st century during adolescence.

Further to this, becoming an adult with a Fontan circulation will bring about another new phase of monitoring, treatments and maintenance of body organs and function. The challenge is lifelong, life-rewarding and of course, not impossible.

Over the past 50 years of Fontan surgery, we have learned about some of the long-term issues of this unique circulation within the body. Some of these include:

- Circulatory failure
- Ventricular dysfunction
- Atrioventricular valve regurgitation
- Arrhythmia
- Protein losing enteropathy (PLE), plastic bronchitis
- Abnormalities in body composition, bone structure and growth
- Liver fibrosis
- Renal dysfunction
- Cognitive, neuropsychological and behavioural deficits.

CONCLUSION AND A LIFELONG COMMITMENT TO YOUR BABY AND THEIR CHD

However, these are all a long way off and "just for today", we are focusing on the situation you find yourself in at present.

The words contained in the previous chapters were my experience. I hope these have been useful in some way. I am an Australian mum and this was my Aussie experience – I cannot speak for the differences between other countries and the way they conduct their "Fontan Dance", or other states within Australia or even other hospitals. But I acknowledge that whichever country you hail from, Fontan surgery is a lifesaving option for your baby and your experience may be similar to mine, and my son's and my family's. The biggest challenge for me while compiling this "guidebook" was keeping the emotion out of the chapters and sticking to the facts to enable you to benefit from my experience. I hope I have achieved this. It is my aim to publish Daniel's unique journey once this book is complete and available. My second book may give you an insider's view of our experience, warts and all. Keep an eye on my website for the launch of my second book www.halfaheart.com.au.

My son Daniel was born at Westmead Public Hospital in Sydney. Very soon after birth, Daniel was transferred to the Children's Hospital Westmead where he received the best care we could have ever asked for, on every occasion for every surgery. There were plenty of setbacks.

The first twelve months of Daniel's life were by far the most demanding and challenging. He was unwell on-and-off and life was tough-going in many respects, especially when his oxygen saturations were in the mid-70s (apparently nothing to worry about they said)! These days he saturates in the high 90s. Nonetheless, Daniel grew, ate and thrived as best as he could manage. Living and breathing was an effort at times but the little champion proved those early professionals very wrong given they told me he wouldn't make 40 weeks. What a champ and a little inspiration. His life every single day reminds us of how lucky we are and how very grateful we remain.

Acknowledgement of Daniel's Team

It is with deepest sincerity that we thank Doctor Stephen Cooper, our cardiologist, who will remain (for as long as he continues to practice and show up for work) the conductor of Daniel's heart.

Daniel had two surgeons – Professor Richard Chard who performed the first two surgeries and laid the foundation for the great Professor David Winlaw to complete Daniel's Fontan and finally provide him with a much better life. What wonderful and talented men. I will love you all forever for the hard work and challenge that you appeared to meet.

At our local level, an absolute legend and champion of a man, paediatrician Doctor Tim McDonald kept a close eye on Daniel every step of the way until his Fontan completion. Doctor Tim brought great relief (to both Daniel and me) every single time that Daniel was hospitalised. The great man would race across to the Canberra Hospital to provide instructions and care to Daniel and the nursing team, all the while communicating with Doctor Cooper. Thanks Tim and go the Wallabies!

For the first few years of Daniel's life, a local GP showed great care and interest in this special little boy. Doctor Mossarif Hossain deserves a mention for the care and time he took in examining Daniel upon each visit (and not restricted to just his precious heart). Thank you doctor.

Last but by no means least is the wonderful, loving, caring, talented and amazing Doctor Catherine (Cate) McDonald, Daniel's osteopath. Cate continues to provide osteopathy to Daniel and has done so religiously, even prior to his birth. We don't have words Doc to thank you for the relief that you have brought to Daniel's system and the maintenance that you continue to provide.

There were so many nurses who assisted along the way and other staff members who worked above and beyond their paid roles. Nicole was Daniel's first ever nurse on the Ward at CHW – she will always be appreciated and precious to us all. Karen Leclair and Glenda Fleming were absolute champions on the nursing and education front. I could not list and thank all of the wonderful humans called nurses that helped us along this journey. God bless you all.

In closing, I sincerely wish you all the best for the journey that lies ahead. I hope it goes as smoothly as possible. I can only encourage you to do what feels right for yourself and your family. My own son Daniel is proof that this life-saving technique works, in the short term anyway.

Long-term, the pressure that the Fontan circulation places on the entire body is challenging but such is life. I do believe that these children are sent to us for a reason. I haven't yet met a child surviving with a CHD who isn't a brave and courageous human who refuses to take no for an answer. They are fighters and they are tough. They teach us about life and bring challenges never experienced before.

Daniel has brought to my own life a joy that cannot be described in words. I am so proud of him and his determination to live that encourages me in new ways too (hence the reason behind this book). His life took our family to undiscovered places and we all survived too. I wish you all the best. Good luck.

Lib.

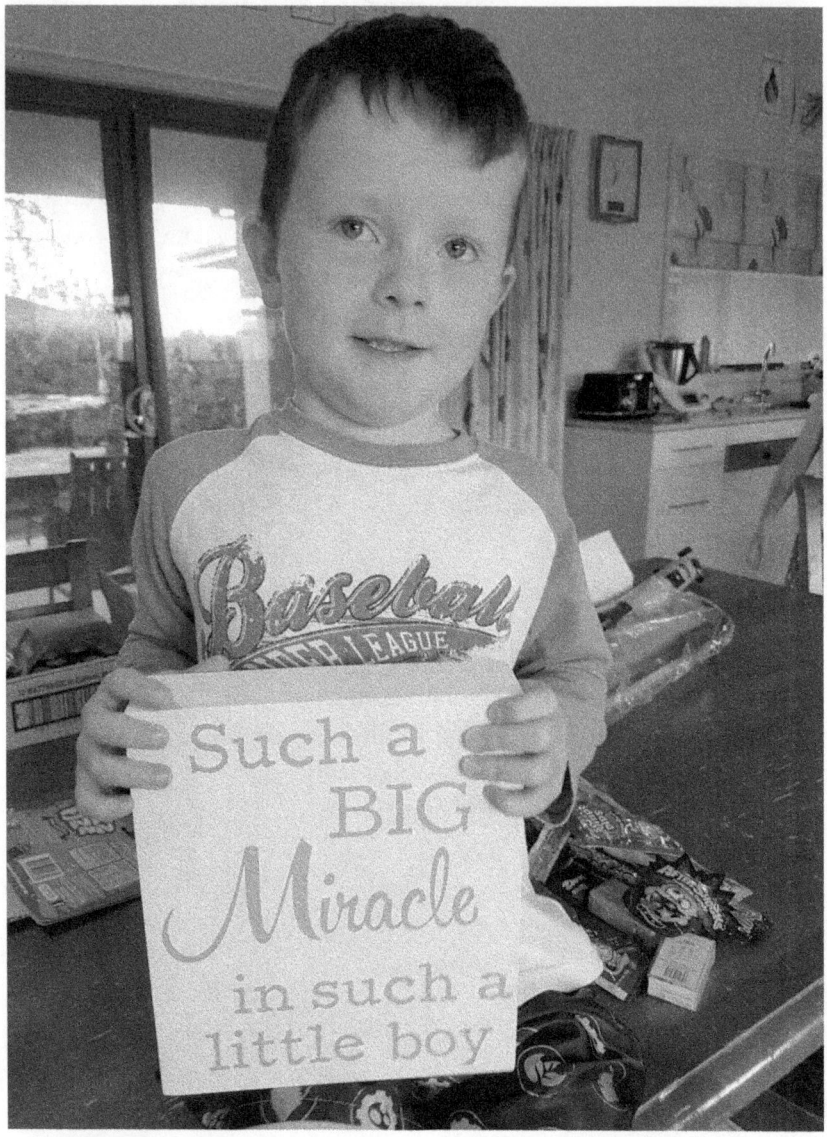

Daniel's 1st Christmas with his Fontan circulation & a whole new life!

RETREAT PAGES

Some of my favourite quotes:

A person is a person, no matter how small.
Dr Seuss, in "Horton Hears a Who".

Courage doesn't always roar. Sometimes courage is the quiet voice at the end of the day saying "I'll try again tomorrow".
Mary Anne Radmacher

On and on you will hike, and I know you'll hike far, and face up to your problems, whatever they are.
Dr Seuss, in "Oh the Places You'll Go".

The best and most beautiful things in the world cannot be seen or even touched, they must be felt with the heart.
Helen Keller

Start doing what is necessary, then do what's possible; and suddenly you are doing the impossible.
> **St Francis of Assisi**

You have brains in your head, you have feet in your shoes, you can steer yourself in any direction you choose.
> **Dr Seuss, in "Oh the Places You'll Go".**

I cannot change the direction of the wind but I can adjust my sails to reach my destination.
> **Jimmy Dean**

The best preparation for tomorrow is doing your best today.
> **H. Jackson Brown Jnr.**

When you reach the end of your rope, tie a knot in it and hang on.
> **Franklin D. Roosevelt**

The only journey is the one within.
> **Rainer Maria Rilkie**

Nothing can dim the light which shines from within.
> **Maya Angelou**

RETREAT PAGES

Think powerfully, positively and confidently. Once I knew only darkness and silence – before my heart leaped to the rapture of living. Your life will unfold for you as you expect it to.

Helen Keller

Piglet noticed that even though he had a very small heart, it could hold a rather large amount of gratitude.

A.A. Milne

The thing that is really hard and really amazing, is giving up on being perfect and beginning the work of becoming yourself.

Anna Quindlen

Our greatest weakness lies in giving up. The most certain way to succeed is always to try just one more time.

Thomas A. Edison

It doesn't matter how slowly you go as long as you do not stop.

Confucius

It always seems impossible until it's done.

Nelson Mandela

With the new day comes new strength and new thoughts.
Eleanor Roosevelt

The journey of a thousand miles begins with one step.
Lao Tzu

When we are no longer able to change a situation, we are challenged to change ourselves.
Victor E. Frankl

The only true wisdom is knowing you know nothing.
Socrates

Where there is love there is life.
Mahatma Ghandi

It is during our darkest moments that we must focus to see the light.
Aristotle

You are greater than you know.
Mother Teresa

Here is my secret, a very simple secret; it is only with the heart that one can see rightly. What is essential is invisible to the eye.

"The Little Prince"
Antoine De Saint Exupery

Some of my favourite prayers:

The Serenity Prayer

God grant me the serenity to accept the things I cannot change, courage to change the things I can and wisdom to know the difference.

St Therese of Lisieux

The loveliest
masterpiece of
the heart of God
is the heart of
a mother.

God's Love

No matter how serious the problems, God's love is greater.
No matter how desperate the situation, God's love is stronger.
Put your trust in Him, for nothing is surer than the power of God's love.

A Prayer for Today

Every day I need you Lord, but this day especially, I need some extra strength to face whatever is to be. This day, more than any day, I need to feel you near, to fortify my courage and to overcome my fear.

By myself I cannot meet the challenge of the hour. There are times when human creatures need a Higher Power, to help them bear what must be borne. And so dear Lord, I pray, hold onto my trembling hand and be with me today.

A Prayer to Saint Anthony of Padua

When I am depressed, help me find hope. When I feel alone, help me find love. When I can't see God anywhere, help me find faith. When I am afraid, help me find trust. When I am weak, help me find courage. When I am sick, help me find healing. When I am overcome by grief, help me find comfort. When I am angry, help me to let go. When I am in trouble, help me find God.
We ask this through Jesus our Lord, Amen.

Don't Quit

When things go wrong as they sometimes will, when the road you're trudging seems all uphill,
When the funds are low and the debts are high and you want to smile but you have to sigh,
When care is pressing you down a bit, rest if you must, but don't you quit.
Life is queer with its twists and turns, as everyone of us sometimes learns
And many a failure turns about, when he might have won, had he stuck it out;
Don't give up though the pace seems slow, you may succeed with another blow,
Success is failure turned inside out, the silver tint of the clouds of doubt,
And you never can tell how close you are, it may be near when it seems so far;
So stick to the fight when you're hardest hit, it's when things seem worst
That you must not quit.

Anon

RETREAT PAGES

Let nothing disturb thee,
Nothing affright thee
All things are passing;
God never changeth;
Patient endurance
Attaineth to all things;
Who God possesseth
In nothing is wanting;
God alone sufficeth.
St Teresa of Avila

Remember, we are all but travellers here
St Mary MacKillop

Listen to the MUSTN'TS
A poem by Shel Silverstein

Listen to the MUSTN'TS, child,
Listen to the DON'TS
Listen to the SHOULDN'TS
The IMPOSSIBLES, the WON'TS
Listen to the NEVER HAVES
Then listen close to me-
Anything can happen, child,
ANYTHING can be

GLOSSARY

Amniocentesis: IS A PROCEDURE whereby amniotic fluid is removed from the uterus for testing. Amniotic fluid is the fluid that surrounds and protects a baby during pregnancy. This fluid contains fetal cells and various proteins. The testing can reveal useful information about the developing fetus.

Cardiologist: a doctor who specialises in the study or treatment of heart diseases and heart abnormalities. In my experience, they are all unique, gifted and talented humans.

Collostrum: known colloquially as "first milk" is produced in the glands of the breast. It can be expressed by hand prior to giving birth (stored and frozen for baby) and is also available immediately following delivery of the newborn.

Cyanosis: a bluish, pinkish or purple discoloration of the skin. This is caused by inadequate oxygenation of the blood or poor circulation.

ECG: an electrocardiogram is a medical test that detects heart problems by measuring the electrical activity generated by the heart as it contracts. It is a safe and non-invasive procedure causing zero pain.

Echocardiogram (echo) an ultrasound of the heart, using high-frequency sound waves to produce various images. Your cardiologist will be looking at the chambers of your baby's heart during the echo, including the size of the heart, heart function, heartbeat, pressures and valves. During an echo you can also listen to the sound of the heart beating and see many images on the monitor including the red and blue blood on the screen.

Fontan: is a palliative procedure conducted on hearts that are deemed impossible to cure.

Neonatal intensive care unit (NICU): usually for newborn babies up to four weeks of age.

Osteopath: in Australia, osteopaths are government registered allied health practitioners who complete university training in anatomy, physiology, pathology, general healthcare diagnosis, and osteopathic techniques. Osteopathy is a drug-free, non-invasive manual therapy that aims to improve health across all body systems by manipulating and strengthening the musculoskeletal framework.

Paediatrician: a doctor who specialises in children and their diseases. He or she may become the "go between" of your general practitioner and cardiologist.

Paediatric intensive care unit (PICU): usually for older babies, toddlers, teens and anyone eligible for Children's Hospital.

Sonographer: person who specialises in the use of ultrasonic imaging devices to produce a range of data. This person will usually perform your ultrasound whilst pregnant.

Surgeon: is the highly trained doctor who will perform the three stages of surgery on your journey to Fontan circulation. He or she will usually specialise in surgical procedures of the heart, at minimum.

ABOUT THE AUTHOR

LIBBY ANDREW IS A stay at home mum based in Canberra, Australia. She has spent the past 10 years running from hospitals, to parks, the supermarket, local schools and the nearby catholic church. Prior to motherhood, Libby spent over 10 years travelling in the Northern Territory of Australia and working in various remote policing roles, from operational police Constable through to Brevet Sergeant. She spent 7 years working in the bush and has a love for the outdoors and our Australian Indigenous tribes.

As a younger adult, Libby spent 10 years chasing a rugby union football and played in the National Women's Rugby Union Team, called the Wallaroos. She played open side flanker and later as hooker in two Women's Rugby World Cups (Holland in 1998 and Spain in 2002), four Hong Kong 7s Tournaments for Aussie Gold and too many other fun-filled sporting commitments to list.

Libby hails from a large family of seven children and two wonderful loving and living parents. She currently lives with her four young sons John, Matthew, Stuart and Daniel and is passionate about life and those she loves. She enjoys travel, the beach and bush walking.

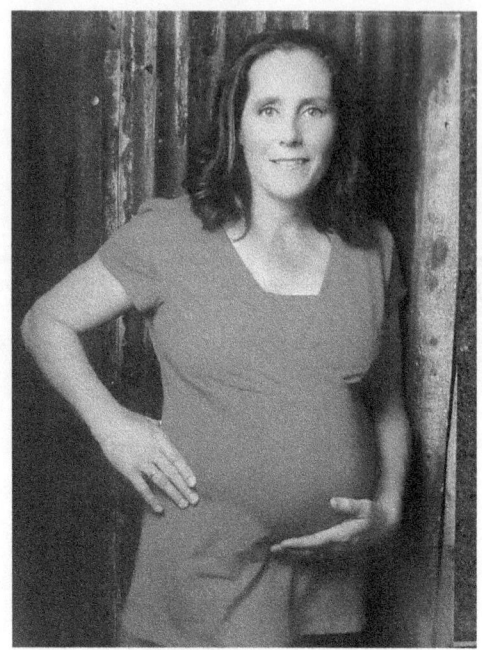

Lib @39 weeks pregnant

ACKNOWLEDGEMENTS

Thanks to my dear Mum and Dad, not only for the proofreading of this book but for everything you have both done for me.

Mylie Sell for your encouragement and help with all of my ideas for this book.

My four sons: John, Matthew, Stuart and Daniel for your lives and the love that we share.

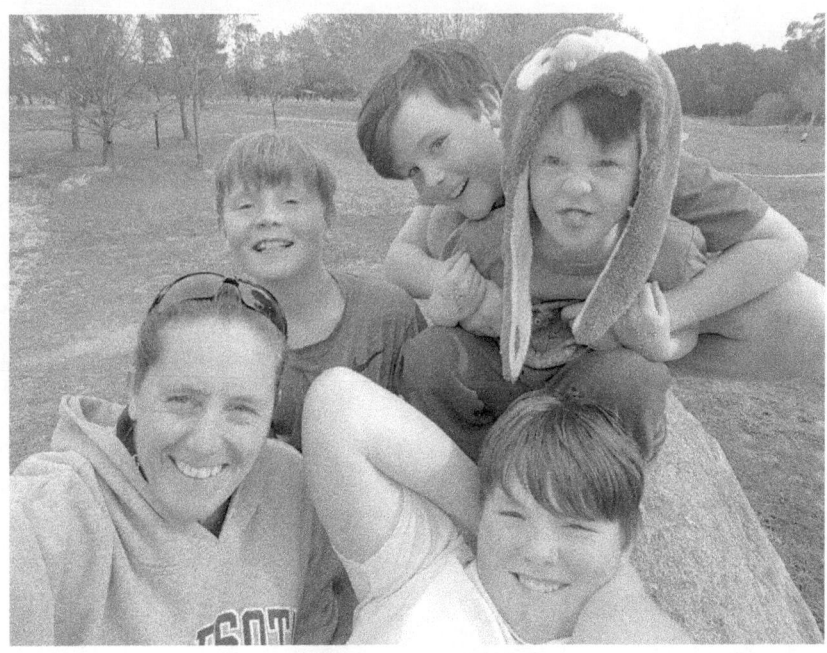

My 4 beautiful boys and I

"HALF A HEART" FACEBOOK GROUP

Join my private Facebook group for updates on this book and other resources. Interact with other parents facing the challenges of CHD in a safe and non-judgemental environment. Read other posts of interest or post your own questions or topics you would like to discuss with me or other members.

Go to Facebook to join this exclusive group.

www.ingramcontent.com/pod-product-compliance
Lightning Source LLC
Chambersburg PA
CBHW031157020426
42333CB00013B/705